Health Care for Underserved Women

Editor

WANDA KAY NICHOLSON

OBSTETRICS AND GYNECOLOGY CLINICS OF NORTH AMERICA

www.obgyn.theclinics.com

Consulting Editor
WILLIAM F. RAYBURN

March 2017 • Volume 44 • Number 1

ELSEVIER

1600 John F. Kennedy Boulevard • Suite 1800 • Philadelphia, Pennsylvania, 19103-2899

http://www.theclinics.com

OBSTETRICS AND GYNECOLOGY CLINICS OF NORTH AMERICA Volume 44, Number 1
March 2017 ISSN 0889-8545, ISBN-13: 978-0-323-50982-4

Editor: Kerry Holland
Developmental Editor: Kristen Helm

Obstetrics and Gynecology Clinics (ISSN 0889-8545) is published quarterly by Elsevier Inc., 360 Park Avenue South, New York, NY 10010-1710. Months of issue are March, June, September, and December. Periodicals postage paid at New York, NY, and additional mailing offices. Subscription price per year is $301.00 (US individuals), $627.00 (US institutions), $100.00 (US students), $377.00 (Canadian individuals), $792.00 (Canadian institutions), $225.00 (Canadian students), $459.00 (international individuals), $792.00 (international institutions), and $225.00 (international students). To receive student/resident rate, orders must be accompanied by name of affiliated institution, date of term, and the signature of program/residency coordinator on institution letterhead. Orders will be billed at individual rate until proof of status is received. Foreign air speed delivery is included in all *Clinics* subscription prices. All prices are subject to change without notice. POSTMASTER: Send address changes to *Obstetrics and Gynecology Clinics*, Elsevier Health Sciences Division, Subscription Customer Service, 3251 Riverport Lane, Maryland Heights, MO 63043. **Customer Service: Telephone: 1-800-654-2452 (U.S. and Canada); 314-447-8871 (outside U.S. and Canada). Fax: 314-447-8029. E-mail: journalscustomerservice-usa@elsevier.com (for print support); journalsonlinesupport-usa@elsevier. com (for online support).**

Reprints. For copies of 100 or more of articles in this publication, please contact the Commercial Reprints Department, Elsevier Inc., 360 Park Avenue South, New York, New York 10010-1710. Tel.: 212-633-3874; Fax: 212-633-3820; E-mail: reprints@elsevier.com.

Obstetrics and Gynecology Clinics of North America is also published in Spanish by McGraw-Hill Interamericana Editores S.A., P.O. Box 5-237, 06500, Mexico; in Portuguese by Reichmann and Affonso Editores, Rio de Janeiro, Brazil; and in Greek by Paschalidis Medical Publications, Athens, Greece.

Obstetrics and Gynecology Clinics of North America is covered in MEDLINE/PubMed (Index Medicus), Excerpta Medica, Current Concepts/Clinical Medicine, Science Citation Index, BIOSIS, CINAHL, and ISI/BIOMED.

Contributors

CONSULTING EDITOR

WILLIAM F. RAYBURN, MD, MBA
Associate Dean, Continuing Medical Education and Professional Development, Distinguished Professor and Emeritus Chair, Obstetrics and Gynecology, University of New Mexico School of Medicine, Albuquerque, New Mexico

EDITOR

WANDA KAY NICHOLSON, MD, MPH, MBA
Professor, Obstetrics and Gynecology; Director, PoWER-Partnerships for Women's Endocrine and Reproductive Health, Department of Obstetrics and Gynecology, Center for Health Promotion and Disease Prevention, Center for Women's Health Research, University of North Carolina School of Medicine, Chapel Hill, North Carolina

AUTHORS

KESHA BAPTISTE-ROBERTS, PhD, MPH
Assistant Professor, Department of Public Health Analysis, School of Community Health & Policy, Morgan State University, Baltimore, Maryland

ALEXANDER BERGER, MD, MPH
Resident Physician, Department of Obstetrics & Gynecology, Thomas Jefferson University Hospital, Philadelphia, Pennsylvania

ALLISON S. BRYANT, MD, MPH
Assistant Professor and Vice Chair of Quality, Equity and Safety, Department of Obstetrics and Gynecology, Massachusetts General Hospital, Boston, Massachusetts

LORECE V. EDWARDS, DrPH
Associate Professor, Department of Behavioral Health Science, School of Community Health & Policy, Morgan State University, Baltimore, Maryland

EVE ESPEY, MD, MPH
Chair, Department of Obstetrics and Gynecology, University of New Mexico Hospitals, University of New Mexico, Albuquerque, New Mexico

SARAH GOPMAN, MD
Associate Professor, Department of Family and Community Medicine, University of New Mexico, Albuquerque, New Mexico

ELIZABETH A. HOWELL, MD, MPP
Professor, Department of Population Health Science and Policy; Professor & System Vice Chair of Research, Department of Obstetrics, Gynecology, and Reproductive Science, Icahn School of Medicine at Mount Sinai, New York, New York

ANDREA JACKSON, MD, MAS
Assistant Clinical Professor, Department of Obstetrics, Gynecology and Reproductive Sciences, University of California, San Francisco, San Francisco, California

VANESSA L. JACOBY, MD, MAS
Department of Obstetrics, Gynecology and Reproductive Sciences, University of California, San Francisco, San Francisco, California

SHANNON K. LAUGHLIN-TOMMASO, MD, MPH
Departments of Obstetrics & Gynecology and Surgery, Mayo Clinic, Rochester, Minnesota

ANGELA K. LAWSON, PhD
Assistant Professor, Division of Reproductive Endocrinology and Infertility, Department of Obstetrics and Gynecology, Feinberg School of Medicine, Northwestern University, Chicago, Illinois

LAWRENCE LEEMAN, MD, MPH
Professor, Department of Family and Community Medicine; Department of Obstetrics and Gynecology, University of New Mexico, Albuquerque, New Mexico

ERICA E. MARSH, MD, MSCI, FACOG
Associate Professor, Chief, Division of Reproductive Endocrinology and Infertility, Department of Obstetrics and Gynecology, University of Michigan Medical School, Ann Arbor, Michigan

JESSICA E. MORSE, MD, MPH
Assistant Professor, Family Planning Division, Department of Obstetrics and Gynecology, University of North Carolina, Chapel Hill, North Carolina

JOYCE MURUTHI, MD
Chief Resident, Department of Obstetrics and Gynecology, University of New Mexico School of Medicine, Albuquerque, New Mexico

EVAN R. MYERS, MD, MPH
Department of Obstetrics and Gynecology, Duke Clinical Research Institute, Duke University, Durham, North Carolina

WANDA KAY NICHOLSON, MD, MPH, MBA
Professor, Obstetrics and Gynecology; Director, PoWER-Partnerships for Women's Endocrine and Reproductive Health, Department of Obstetrics and Gynecology, Center for Health Promotion and Disease Prevention, Center for Women's Health Research, University of North Carolina School of Medicine, Chapel Hill, North Carolina

EBELE ORANUBA, MBBS, MPH
Research Assistant, Department of Public Health Analysis, School of Community Health & Policy, Morgan State University, Baltimore, Maryland

SHANTHI RAMESH, MD
Fellow, Family Planning Division, Department of Obstetrics and Gynecology, University of North Carolina, Chapel Hill, North Carolina

WILLIAM F. RAYBURN, MD, MBA
Associate Dean, Continuing Medical Education and Professional Development, Distinguished Professor and Emeritus Chair, Obstetrics and Gynecology, University of New Mexico School of Medicine, Albuquerque, New Mexico

JODY STONEHOCKER, MD
Assistant Professor, Department of Obstetrics and Gynecology, University of New Mexico School of Medicine, Albuquerque, New Mexico

MARY BETH SUTTER, MD
Assistant Professor, Department of Family and Community Medicine, University of New Mexico, Albuquerque, New Mexico

LAUREN THAXTON, MD, MBA
Fellow in Family Planning, Department of Obstetrics and Gynecology, University of New Mexico Hospitals, University of New Mexico, Albuquerque, New Mexico

NIYA WERTS, PhD, MIS
Associate Professor, Department of Health Science, Towson University, Baltimore, Maryland

SARAHN M. WHEELER, MD
Assistant Professor of Maternal Fetal Medicine, Department of Obstetrics and Gynecology, Duke University Medical Center, Durham, North Carolina

JENNIFER ZEITLIN, DSc, MA
Adjunct Faculty, Department of Population Health Science and Policy, Icahn School of Medicine at Mount Sinai, New York, New York; Research Director, Inserm UMR 1153, Obstetrical, Perinatal and Pediatric Epidemiology Research Team (Epopé), Center for Epidemiology and Biostatistics Sorbonne Paris Cité, DHU Risks in pregnancy, Paris Descartes University, Paris, France

Contents

Foreword: Reducing Barriers to Invest in Improved Health Care   xi

William F. Rayburn

Preface: Multilevel Barriers to Optimizing Care in Underserved Women   xiii

Wanda Kay Nicholson

Racial and Ethnic Disparities in Health and Health Care   1

Sarahn M. Wheeler and Allison S. Bryant

A health disparity is defined as an increased burden of an adverse health outcome or health determinant within a specific subset of the population. There are well-documented racial and ethnic disparities throughout health care at the patient, provider, and health care system levels. As the minority populations within the United States grow to record numbers, it is increasingly important to invest in efforts to characterize, understand, and end racial and ethnic disparities in health care. Inequities in health outcomes and care pose real threats to the entire nation's well-being. Eliminating health disparities is fundamental to the well-being, productivity, and viability of the entire nation.

Quality of Care and Disparities in Obstetrics   13

Elizabeth A. Howell and Jennifer Zeitlin

Growing attention is being paid to obstetric quality of care as patients are pressing the health care system to measure and improve quality. There is also an increasing recognition of persistent racial and ethnic disparities prevalent in obstetric outcomes. Yet few studies have linked obstetric quality of care with racial and ethnic disparities. This article reviews definitions of quality of care, health disparities, and health equity as they relate to obstetric care and outcomes; describes current efforts and challenges in obstetric quality measurement; and proposes 3 steps in an effort to develop, track, and improve quality and reduce disparities in obstetrics.

Reassessing Unintended Pregnancy: Toward a Patient-centered Approach to Family Planning   27

Jessica E. Morse, Shanthi Ramesh, and Andrea Jackson

Underserved women, especially those with low incomes and from racial and ethnic minorities, experience a disproportionate share of unintended pregnancies in the United States. Although unintended pregnancy rates are general markers of women's health and status, they may not accurately capture women's experiences of these pregnancies or their social circumstances. A patient-centered approach to family planning optimizes women's reproductive preferences, is cognizant of historical harms and current disparities, and may more comprehensively address the issue of unintended pregnancy. Clinicians, researchers, and policy makers can all adopt a patient-centered approach to help underserved women regain their reproductive autonomy.

Family Planning American Style Redux: Unintended Pregnancy Improves, Barriers Remain   **41**

Lauren Thaxton and Eve Espey

This article discusses barriers to reducing unintended pregnancy. Numerous factors may explain the high rate of unintended pregnancy in the United States, including inadequate sex education, confusing media messages about sex, cultural attitudes about sex and young parenting, conflation of contraception with abortion, inadequate health care access, burdensome contraceptive dispensing practices, and hospital merger limitations on care. Successful and promising approaches to expanding access to reproductive health care and reducing unintended pregnancy are discussed.

Leveraging Opportunities for Postpartum Weight Interventions   **57**

Alexander Berger and Wanda Kay Nicholson

Approximately 20 million US women are considered overweight or obese. African American women share a disproportionate burden of obesity. To date, few studies have assessed the effects of behavioral interventions, tailored to the specific lifestyle challenges of postpartum African American women. Efforts to address the disparate rates of obesity in African American women should include assessment of knowledge and knowledge gaps, development and testing of behavioral interventions, and translation of evidence into clinical practice. Developing interventions that are tailored to this vulnerable group of women and promoting policies that can begin to address the health consequences in African American women is a public health priority.

Addressing Health Care Disparities Among Sexual Minorities   **71**

Kesha Baptiste-Roberts, Ebele Oranuba, Niya Werts, and Lorece V. Edwards

There is evidence of health disparities between sexual minority and heterosexual populations. Although the focus of lesbian, gay, bisexual, and transgender health research has been human immunodeficiency virus/acquired immunodeficiency syndrome and sexually transmitted infection among men who have sex with men, there are health disparities among sexual minority women. Using the minority stress framework, these disparities may in part be caused by individual prejudice, social stigma, and discrimination. To ensure equitable health for all, there is urgent need for targeted culturally sensitive health promotion, cultural sensitivity training for health care providers, and intervention-focused research.

Disparities in Fibroid Incidence, Prognosis, and Management   **81**

Shannon K. Laughlin-Tommaso, Vanessa L. Jacoby, and Evan R. Myers

Health disparities in fibroid prevalence, prognosis, and treatment exist for underserved women. Access to fibroid treatment alternatives can have significant effect on choices and outcomes of fibroid disease.

Patient-centered Care to Address Barriers for Pregnant Women with Opioid Dependence   95

Mary Beth Sutter, Sarah Gopman, and Lawrence Leeman

> Pregnant women affected by substance use often encounter barriers to treatment, including housing insecurity, poverty, mental health issues, social stigma, and access to health care. Providers may lack the resources needed to provide quality care. Clinicians offering prenatal care to women with substance use disorder are encouraged to support family-centered, multidisciplinary care to women and their infants, focusing on harm reduction. Collaboration between providers of maternity care, substance abuse treatment, case management, family primary care, and pediatric developmental care can improve outcomes during pregnancy and through the early years of parenting.

Hearing the Silenced Voices of Underserved Women: The Role of Qualitative Research in Gynecologic and Reproductive Care   109

Angela K. Lawson and Erica E. Marsh

> In order to provide effective evidence-based health care to women, rigorous research that examines women's lived experiences in their own voices is needed. However, clinical health research has often excluded the experiences of women and minority patient populations. Further, clinical research has often relied on quantitative research strategies; this provides an interesting but limited understanding of women's health experiences and hinders the provision of effective patient-centered care. This article defines qualitative research and its unique contributions to research, and provides examples of how qualitative research has given insights into the reproductive health perspectives and behaviors of underserved women.

Is There a Shortage of Obstetrician-Gynecologists?   121

Jody Stonehocker, Joyce Muruthi, and William F. Rayburn

> Projections of supply and demand for obstetricians-gynecologists suggest a current minimal or modest shortage that will worsen in the future. The US adult female population is expected to increase by more than 20% by 2045 and represents a key driver for increased demand for health care services. The annual number of obstetrician-gynecologists (ob-gyn) residency graduates has increased negligibly, whereas the proportion accepted into fellowships increased steadily, reducing those in general practice. The gradual increase in proportion of ob-gyns who are women coincides with desires for more work-life balance and earlier retirement from clinical practice. As the supply of advanced practice providers of women's health services grows, the need for more ob-gyns could be less to meet the projected demand.

Index   133

OBSTETRICS AND GYNECOLOGY CLINICS

FORTHCOMING ISSUES

June 2017
Obstetrics and Gynecology: Maintenance of Knowledge
Janice L. Bacon and Paul G. Tomich, *Editors*

September 2017
Evaluation and Management of Vulvar Disease
Aruna Venkatesan, *Editor*

December 2017
Management of Labor and Delivery
Aaron B. Caughey, *Editor*

RECENT ISSUES

December 2016
Critical Care Obstetrics for the Obstetrician and Gynecologist
Carolyn M. Zelop and Stephanie R. Martin, *Editors*

September 2016
Hysterectomy and the Alternatives
John A. Occhino and Emanuel C. Trabuco, *Editors*

June 2016
Primary Care of Adult Women
James N. Woodruff and Anita K. Blanchard, *Editors*

Foreword
Reducing Barriers to Invest in Improved Health Care

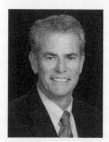

William F. Rayburn, MD, MBA
Consulting Editor

This issue of *Obstetrics and Gynecology Clinics of North America*, edited by Wanda Nicholson, MD, deals with special considerations surrounding the health care of underserved women. These persons are vulnerable, since they are unable to obtain quality health care by virtue of barriers created by poverty, race, or ethnicity disparities, cultural differences, geography, sexual orientation, gender identity, disabilities, or other factors that contribute to health care inequities.

Underserved women are often in need of more health services because of higher rates of chronic conditions and unmet reproductive health care needs. Understanding issues important to underserved populations is critical from a health care system perspective. A well-functioning system responds in a balanced way to any population's needs and expectations by improving the health status of individuals and their communities; defending against health threats; protecting against the financial consequences of ill health; providing equitable access to patient-centered care; and ensuring patient participation in their health decision making.

As described in this issue, underserved women are at increased risk of health problems related to limited access to quality care. Higher costs disproportionately affect women with low incomes and minority women, and more than half report delaying or avoiding needed care due to cost. Some experience challenges in receiving coverage for critical services, such as contraception and comprehensive maternity care. In addition, the challenges may not be due to their lack of insurance or inadequate coverage alone, but to any combination of educational, cultural, social isolation, and logistical factors.

Passage of the Patient Protection and Affordable Care Act brought promise of increased health insurance coverage for underserved women. Regardless of future modifications, this law permitted direct access to obstetrician-gynecologists, which would facilitate women's health care delivery. This issue deals with several issues affecting the health of underserved women: preconception care, well-woman visits,

Obstet Gynecol Clin N Am 44 (2017) xi–xii
http://dx.doi.org/10.1016/j.ogc.2016.12.002
0889-8545/17/© 2016 Published by Elsevier Inc.

contraception, mental health care, opioid dependence, premalignant and malignant conditions, and comprehensive maternity care before and after delivery. A central theme in this issue is that quality care depends on appropriately trained and certified health care providers, open communication and transparency, ongoing performance evaluations of providers, use of evidence-based guidelines, and patient education.

This issue also introduces the reader to another topic of interest, "Is there a shortage of obstetrician-gynecologists?," that complements the main theme of this issue. This question, raised by Drs Stonehocker, Muruthi, and Rayburn, is timely, since the number of residents being trained has increased minimally. The adult female population in the United States continues to grow, and more residency graduates are electing to undertake subspecialty fellowship training. The impending shortage of obstetrician-gynecologists in general practice will require a team-based approach with non-physician providers in caring for underserved women.

A special thanks goes to the many authors who contributed to this issue. They advocate for underserved women in the following key areas: providing culturally competent care; tracking outcomes; coordinating key services such as mental health and reproductive health; and funding quantitative and qualitative research to develop effective interventions. Their effort and dedication to hearing the silenced voices of underserved women are much appreciated.

William F. Rayburn, MD, MBA
Continuing Medical Education & Professional Development
MSC10 5580, 1 University of New Mexico
Albuquerque, NM 87131-0001, USA

E-mail address:
wrayburn@salud.unm.edu

Preface

Multilevel Barriers to Optimizing Care in Underserved Women

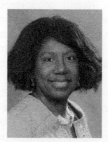

Wanda Kay Nicholson, MD, MPH, MBA
Editor

We are delighted to devote this issue of *Obstetrics and Gynecology Clinics of North America* to the topic of Underserved Women. It is crucial that clinicians, health policy-makers, and community health leaders acknowledge the broad and diverse population of women within the United States. As shown in **Fig. 1**, the term "Underserved Women" does not apply simply to women of a certain racial/ethnic group or socioeconomic level. Rather, the term "Underserved Women" refers to any group of women

Fig. 1. Topics related to underserved women and barriers to optimizing care. CVD, cardiovascular disease.

Obstet Gynecol Clin N Am 44 (2017) xiii–xv
http://dx.doi.org/10.1016/j.ogc.2016.12.001
0889-8545/17/© 2016 Published by Elsevier Inc.

obgyn.theclinics.com

who have limited access to services due to personal, geographic, provider, or health system barriers. Such barriers decrease the availability of health services to optimize physical, mental, and emotional well-being.

The current health care environment is challenging, for both patients and the clinicians who are dedicated to providing care. Despite advances in medications, procedures, therapies, contraception, and neonatal care, disparities in health outcomes traverse social, educational, geographic, and racial strata. Efforts to address disparities in access to care and health outcomes must begin with engaging multiple stakeholders (ie, patients, clinicians, health policy leaders, health organizations) in meaningful conversations to address multilevel barriers, such as personal, provider-based, health system, and community level barriers, to optimize health care and achieve equity in obstetric and gynecologic outcomes. To this end, we provide a concise body of reviews to bring further attention to multilevel barriers and solutions to address underserved women.

We begin with a discussion of racial/ethnic disparities in health and health care, focusing on disparities in disease conditions and the implicit and explicit biases that can contribute to disparities in access and delivery of health care services to improve these conditions. Next, the development and implementation of perinatal quality indicators to improve birth equity are discussed. While access to effective contraceptive methods has improved, we discuss a framework for patient-centered reproductive life planning to reduce disparities in unintended pregnancies as well as lingering barriers to reproductive choice in the United States. We provide an evidence-focused review of weight-loss interventions in the postpartum period and current initiatives to implement programs for healthy living to women living in varied communities. The pressing need to better identify and provide solutions to health care disparities among minority lesbian, gay, bisexual, and transgender individuals has been highlighted by state and federal agencies, including the National Institute of Minority Health Disparities. We discuss efforts to improve health outcomes through community-level interventions. While national efforts are focused on the comparative effectiveness of surgical treatments for uterine fibroids, we discuss the limited access to surgical treatments experienced by racial/ethnic groups of women who suffer disproportionately from uterine fibroids and women living in certain geographical regions. It is estimated that in 2013 to 2014, 5.3% of women aged 15 to 44 were using illicit drugs during pregnancy. We discuss family-centered approaches to care for women and their infants that enhance the mother-child dyad and focus on harm reduction. We conclude with an article on qualitative methods. A key step in addressing the needs of underserved women is providing a pathway by which they are able to voice their needs, perspectives, and preferences of care. Qualitative methods provide a reasonable and substantive parallel to traditional quantitative methods, such as observational studies and clinical trials, that allow patients to talk about the health care topics that are most important to them and best meet their needs. We also broadly speak to the access of obstetrician-gynecologists and current workforce capacity.

Our hope is that this issue provides readers with a transdisciplinary perspective on the multilevel challenges and potential solutions to meet the health care needs of underserved women. In addition, this issue is a call to action for obstetricians and gynecologists to continue to be an active voice for underserved women across the United States. Most importantly, we hope that this body of work re-emphasizes that underserved women are any group of women in which access to or provision of care has not been fully optimized.

Wanda Kay Nicholson, MD, MPH, MBA
PoWER-Partnerships for Women's
Endocrine and Reproductive Health
Department of Obstetrics and Gynecology
Center for Health Promotion and Disease Prevention
Center for Women's Health Research
University of North Carolina School of Medicine
University of North Carolina
3027 Old Clinic Building, CB 7570
Chapel Hill, NC 27599-7570, USA

E-mail address:
wknichol@med.unc.edu

Racial and Ethnic Disparities in Health and Health Care

Sarahn M. Wheeler, MD[a],*, Allison S. Bryant, MD, MPH[b]

KEYWORDS

• Race • Ethnicity • Disparities • Health care • Inequity

KEY POINTS

- Racial and ethnic disparities exist on every level of health care system: the patient, the provider, and the health care system.
- On the patient level, genetic predispositions to inherited conditions that cluster within race groups and shared cultural beliefs within ethnic groups are important mediators of disparities.
- Providers, even though most often well meaning, are subject to implicit biases that can have a negative impact on interactions with minority patients and contribute to disparities.
- Although there are improvements in access to care for racial and ethnic minorities, there remains room for improvements to improve disparities at the health care system level.
- Research dedicated to characterizing, understanding, and ending racial and ethnic disparities in health care is urgently needed.

INTRODUCTION: DEFINING HEALTH DISPARITIES AND THE NATIONAL IMPACT

Few topics generate greater controversy than issues of race and ethnicity in the United States. *Race* — a categorization based on common physical characteristics — and *ethnicity* — a categorization based on shared cultural traits — both have a powerful impact on one's experience in America. Disparities in health care present notable examples of the intersection between race, ethnicity, and the American experience. A *health disparity* is defined as an increased burden of an adverse health outcome or health determinant within a specific subset of the population.[1] Health disparities can and do affect many different groups; however, there is a long-standing history of disparities affecting racial and ethnic minorities in the United States.

Disclosure Statement: The authors have nothing to disclose.
[a] Department of Obstetrics and Gynecology, Duke University Medical Center, 2608 Erwin Road, Durham, NC 27705, USA; [b] Department of Obstetrics and Gynecology, Massachusetts General Hospital, 55 Fruit Street, Founders 4, Boston, MA 02114, USA
* Corresponding author.
E-mail address: sarahn.wheeler@duke.edu

Obstet Gynecol Clin N Am 44 (2017) 1–11
http://dx.doi.org/10.1016/j.ogc.2016.10.001
0889-8545/17/© 2016 Elsevier Inc. All rights reserved.

Although from a biological standpoint there are far more similarities between racial and ethnic groups than there are differences,[2] notable differences in outcomes along these primarily socially constructed lines are impossible to ignore. In 2013, the Centers for Disease Control and Prevention reported an average life expectancy of 79.1 years for whites and 75.5 years for blacks.[3] Although this 3-year gap represents an improvement in the life expectancy disparity, which was as high as 15 years at the start of the twentieth century, the scientific community is still in the early stages of understanding the complex causes and implications of disparities along race and ethnic lines.

The distinction between disparities in *health outcomes* and *health care* is worthy of mention. Although differences in prevalence of infant mortality or obesity, for example, are considered disparities in outcome that may have contributions from both inside and outside the health care system, disparities in health care arise distinctly within the health care arena and include such inequities as differential access to care or differences in likelihood of receipt of specific therapies or counseling.

There is mounting interest in research and public policy exploring racial and ethnic disparities because minority populations are growing in the United States. In 2015, the US Census Bureau reported that racial and ethnic minorities comprise 38.4% of the population.[4] It is projected that by 2050 non-Hispanic whites will no longer be the majority group within the United States.[4] With the evolving population demographics, the burden of health and health care disparities is becoming increasingly costly both for the patients who suffer the adverse health affect and the health care system that is ill-equipped to manage the economic effects of these adverse outcomes.

The *Harvard Business Review* estimates the US cost of race and ethnic health disparities to be in excess of $245 billion dollars annually.[5] These costs are directly reflected in health care premiums for employer-based health plans. As an example, it is estimated that if the disparity in effective asthma treatment of African Americans was reduced by only 10%, American workers would save more than $1600 per person on a yearly basis.[5] Additionally, racial and ethnic minorities are known to have increased rates of sexually transmitted infection, unintended pregnancy, and poor pregnancy outcomes, all with far-reaching social and economic effects.[6–11]

The profound economic and social impact of health and health care disparities is notable among minority women who are vulnerable to disparities that affect not only themselves but also their childbearing, children, and, therefore, communities. Obstetrician-gynecologists have a place at the forefront of growing efforts to identify, understand, and narrow these disparate outcomes.

THE ETIOLOGY OF RACIAL AND ETHNIC DISPARITIES IN HEALTH CARE

Social determinants of health, such as income, wealth, and educational and employment opportunities, have effects on health outcomes. Even when controlling for the social determinants that are able to be accurately captured and measured, however, disparities remain.[12] Contributions stemming from multiple levels of health care — from the individual patient to the provider and hospitals to the health care system at large, including the subset that is medical research — all have profound impacts on health disparities.[12] Narrowing outcome gaps requires strategies aimed at improving disparities on each of these levels.

Patient-Level Factors

It is tempting to completely dismiss race and ethnicity as biologically meaningless social constructs with no bearing on medicine beyond their association with social determinants of health. The average proportion of genetic difference between

2 randomly selected humans' DNA is approximately 1 in 1000 nucleotides.[2] In comparison, this is much less than the genetic heterogeneity found between 2 different fruit flies.[2] Even a difference in a single nucleotide, however, can have a profound impact on health, as evidenced by single nucleotide diseases, such as sickle cell anemia, cystic fibrosis, and the thalassemias. The frequency of such single nucleotide polymorphisms is often linked to race and ethnicity because these single nucleotide polymorphisms cluster within groups more likely to share a common region of origin or ancestral lineage. Using race and ethnicity to risk-stratify patients for specific diseases is important to determining whether screening for various conditions is reasonable and cost-effective. Within obstetrics and gynecology, the intersection between race and genetics takes on particular significance. Prenatal screening and diagnostic testing are becoming increasingly available. Although race or ethnicity alone cannot rule in or rule out risk for particular diseases, the American College of Obstetricians and Gynecologists (ACOG) and the Society for Maternal-Fetal Medicine both recommend counseling patients about prenatal genetic screening and testing based on race and ethnicity.[13,14]

The complex history of race and ethnicity in the United States may affect individual patients' responses to medical recommendations for screening tests and adherence to treatment plans, contributing to disparate outcomes along racial lines. There are numerous historical examples of racial and ethnic groups being targeted for forced medical procedures or experimentation. One of the most notorious examples was the Tuskegee Study of Untreated Syphilis in the Negro Male, a 40-year project in which black men with syphilis were observed to determine the natural history of the disease, even after the introduction of penicillin as an efficacious therapy for the illness. Although reparations and a formal apology on behalf of the nation were forthcoming in the 1970s–1990s, the legacy of mistrust of the health care system among many American blacks lingers.[15] Similarly, forced sterilization, often based solely on a women's race or ethnicity, persisted until the 1970s in some US states[16] and victimized countless women. Although the echoes of such atrocities have lasting effects, recent data suggest there is hope for restoring trust within minority communities. In a focus group study exploring physician mistrust, many African Americans participants recounted personal episodes of mistreatment and discrimination. Even in that setting, however, participants reported that physicians can and do earn their trust based on the physicians' perceived competence and communication skills.[17]

Aside from considerations of mistrust, racial and cultural influences on patient values, attitudes, and preferences may affect care that is accepted and received. There are examples of patient preferences related to race, ethnicity and culture throughout health care; however, cultural differences are particularly salient in women's health. Many of the traditions surrounding pregnancy and child-rearing are strongly influenced by race and culture. As an example, black women are 16% less likely to breastfeed and breastfeed for shorter duration compared with white women despite well-documented maternal and child health benefits.[18] Black women may view bottle feeding as preferred because their mothers and grandmothers used this method[19]: the roots of this cultural preference may be linked to disparities in care. Recent studies attempting to unpack this disparity suggest minority women are more likely to deliver in hospitals with poorly developed programs to promote lactation.[18] In a study examining breastfeeding among military women, where quality of care is likely more uniform, the black-white gap in breastfeeding duration was significantly narrower,[20] supporting the notion that the effects of personal and familial attitudes and preferences are often entangled with differentials in access and quality of care.

In the 1990s, McGinnnis and Foege[21] estimated that 40% of mortality — and conversely, health — in the United States was attributable to health behaviors. Certainly, then, disparities in health behaviors at a personal level contribute to disparities in health outcomes. Health behaviors, such as exercise, tobacco use, and nutritious food intake, are inextricably linked with social determinants of health, such as poverty, lower educational attainment, food insecurity, and unsafe built environments.[22–25] That said, these social determinants have significant overlap with race and ethnicity; the contributions of health behaviors to disparities therefore should not be discounted.

Provider-Level Factors

Health care providers are also an important potential source of health care disparities through conscious and unconscious biases toward minority groups. Many providers, nurses, administrators, policy makers, and others involved in health care today lived during times when segregation and open racism was not only acceptable but also legally enforced.[26] Although Jim Crow laws have been removed and most Americans no longer subscribe to blatantly racist rhetoric, even the most well-meaning providers may have subconscious biases that contribute to health disparities and may result in suboptimal interactions with minority patients.[27]

Several studies have documented that providers are less likely to give analgesics to black patients seeking treatment in an emergency department compared with whites.[28–30] Recent work demonstrated prevalent false beliefs among laypeople and medical trainees alike about biological differences in the experience of pain between blacks and whites; among the medical students and residents, these beliefs led to inequitable recommendations for treatment of pain.[31] Additionally, studies have shown black patients with symptoms concerning for acute coronary syndrome were less likely to receive indicated treatments compared with white patients.[32,33] In important work attempting to understand the mechanism of these differential recommendations, Greenwald and colleagues[34] demonstrated that the higher a physician's preference favoring white Americans, as measured by the Implicit Association Test, the lower their likelihood of recommending thrombolysis for black simulated patients with acute coronary syndrome and the higher their likelihood of recommending the same therapy for white patients with identical presentations.[35] Within obstetrics and gynecology, higher cesarean delivery rates and delayed referral for infertility treatments may be, in part, due to implicit provider biases.

Happily, some studies show improvement in implicit bias with physician education and increased awareness of their implicit biases.[35,36] Ongoing education during medical training and continuing postgraduate education about health disparities and implicit bias will be integral to improving disparities in health care.

Health Care System and Institutional Level Factors

Just as many individual providers lived through a time when racial segregation and prejudice was the rule of law, many medical institutions date back to the times of slavery.[37] With only a cursory glance through history, multiple examples of inappropriate medical experimentation and refusal of care for racial and ethnic minorities in routine practice can be identified.[37,38] There is undoubtedly institutionalized discrimination that continues to mar the health care system; however, significant progress is being made.

Perhaps one of the most significant advances in racial and ethnic health disparities is improved health care access, particularly within women's health. Recent data show black women and Hispanic women are equally likely as white women to have had

Papanicolaou smear screening within the past 3 years and a mammogram within the past 2 years. Despite these advancements, black women and Hispanic women are still more likely to die from both breast and cervical cancers compared with white women.[39–42] This paradox highlights that although improvements in access to care and services are critical, this is not the only component to narrowing health care disparities.

Since it became law in 2010, the Affordable Care Act has been the subject of significant controversy in the United States. Political debate aside, it is clear that since the implementation of the health insurance marketplace in 2013, rates of uninsured among racial and ethnic minorities have declined.[43] Despite improvement in access to care, disparities still remain —particularly within quality of care.[43] In the 2015 Agency for Healthcare Research and Quality *National Healthcare Quality and Disparities Report*, 79% of the health care quality disparities indicators were worse or unchanged for Hispanic patients.[43] For black patients, 88% of the quality indicators were worse or unchanged.[43] There is still significant work to be done to uncover, understand, and end the disparities in health care suffered by racial and ethnic minorities.

Research

Evidence-based medicine depends on volunteers who willingly participate in medical research to uncover novel therapies and to compare the efficacy of known therapies. Until recent years, there were limited efforts to ensure underrepresented minorities were offered opportunities to participate in clinical research.[44] It was often assumed that minorities are less interested in research participation due to mistrust of the medical system, limited compliance, and language barriers. Recent data challenge these notions, however, and studies show no difference between whites and minorities in terms of willingness to participate in research.[45] Without data including racial and ethnic minorities, a provider's ability to make high-quality medical recommendations for minority patients is inherently limited. Since the mid-1990s the National Institutes of Health (NIH) has required that researchers maintain gender, race, and ethnicity data on participants.[46] Inclusion of racial and ethnic minorities in medical research is particularly important in light of numerous examples of differences in therapeutic response mediated by race throughout medicine, including obstetrics and gynecology.[47–49] Continuing efforts to broaden the base of culturally competent researchers who actively recruit diverse participant populations are an integral part of realizing a future devoid of racial and ethnic health disparities.

FUTURE DIRECTIONS AND STRATEGIES FOR IMPROVEMENT

In 2015, the ACOG Committee on Health Care for Underserved Women revised a committee opinion, "Racial and Ethnic Disparities in Obstetrics and Gynecology," with recommendations for obstetrician-gynecologists to help end racial and ethnic disparities within their field[50] (**Box 1**). Efforts are under way to improve disparities using these recommendations; however, there is room for new ideas to raise awareness, promote research, diversify the workforce, and educate patients, all with the goal of ending health disparities.

Raising Awareness

In 2000, the Healthy People 2010 goal was to eliminate health disparities by 2010. Although this deadline for this lofty goal has long since come and gone, there has been increasing awareness of heath disparities among medical providers. When

Box 1
American College of Obstetricians and Gynecologists Committee on Health Care for Underserved Women recommendations to address racial and ethnic disparities in obstetrics and gynecology

1. Raising awareness among colleagues, staff, and hospital administrators about the prevalence of racial and ethnic disparities

2. Understanding the role that practitioner bias can play in health outcomes and health disparities

3. Strongly encouraging the adoption of federal standards for the collection of race and ethnicity information in clinical and administrative data to better identify disparities

4. Promoting research that not only identifies structural and cultural barriers to care but also tests the effectiveness of the interventions to address such barriers

5. Educating patients in a culturally sensitive manner about steps they can take to prevent disease conditions more prevalent in their racial and ethnic groups

6. Supporting and assisting in the recruitment of obstetrician gynecologists and other health care providers from racial and ethnic minorities into academic and community health care fields

From Racial and ethnic disparities in obstetrics and gynecology. Committee Opinion No. 649. American College of Obstetricians and Gynecologists. Obstet Gynecol 2015;126:e130–4; with permission.

asked if the health care system treated people unfairly based on an individual's race or ethnicity, approximately 70% of physicians in 2002 responded, "rarely or never." By 2005, fewer than 25% of physicians disagreed with the statement, "minority patients generally receive lower quality care than white patients."[51] Although these queries may not measure exactly the same constructs, it seems likely that targeted awareness campaigns have been successful at reaching providers. Most programs aimed at raising awareness about health disparities are aimed at physicians and nurses; however, it must be acknowledged that the patient experience begins the moment a patient reaches out to seek care and is likely influenced by past experiences with the health care system. Therefore, it is imperative that all medical and support staff, none of whom is immune to explicit and implicit biases, receive training and education about cultural sensitivity and the impact of racial and ethnic disparities in health care.

Promoting Research

Throughout history, there are countless examples of medical research leading to ground-breaking discoveries that eradicate disease and suffering. From the early 1990s to the present day, there has been a steady increase in research and funding dedicated to detecting, understanding, and eliminating racial and ethnic disparities in health care. Intuitively for some, the notion of ending disparities by being color-blind and ignoring differences between racial and ethnic groups is an attractive one. Collecting more detailed racial and ethnic data in research, however, has the potential to uncover disparities and yield innovative solutions to narrow outcome gaps. Until recently, most race data were limited to blacks and white. Efforts lead by the NIH encouraging researchers to gather and report detailed racial and ethnic demographic data are an important step toward this goal; however, there is still significant work to be done. The NIH guidelines currently include 6 race and ethnic categories: white, black or African American, Hispanic or Latino, Asian, American Indian or Alaska Native, and Native Hawaiian or Other Pacific Islander.[52] As more research following these guidelines is published, greater insight into racial and ethnic health disparities will undoubtedly be gained. Additionally, collecting detailed race, ethnicity, and language data as part of standard clinical care, outside of research endeavors, will allow for relevant outcome and care comparisons and can enable improvements in quality of care.

Diversifying the Health Care Workforce and Ensuring Cultural Competence

Despite the growing US minority population, only 9% of physicians and 19% of registered nurses identified as being from a minority group in 2014 and 2013, respectively.[53,54] Although the evidence is not entirely consistent, there are data that suggest that concordance between patients and providers along axes of race, ethnicity, language, and/or social class may improve health care outcomes and patient experiences.[55–58] Efforts to increase diversity within the health care workforce to more accurately reflect the culture and ethnic diversity within the United States have the potential to have a positive impact on the health care system,[59] although it is impractical to consider strategies to end health disparities in the short term solely by matching patients and providers by race and ethnicity. Therefore, promoting knowledge and education to all providers and members of the health care team about disparities and ensuring cultural and linguistic competence among the existing and upcoming health workforce will continue to have a critical role. Much of this work is being promoted at the federal and state levels: in 2000, the Office of Minority Health, within the US Department of Health and Human Services, released the first *National Standards for Culturally and Linguistically Appropriate Services in Health and Health Care*, which developed a framework for health care systems to provide quality and equitable care to diverse populations, which included among the recommendations the recruitment of a diverse workforce, the availability of appropriate interpreter services for those with limited English proficiency, and partnerships with communities to ensure the delivery of culturally appropriate services.[60]

Patient Education

In addition to promoting knowledge and education among medical professionals, it is imperative that the racial and ethnic minority patients at increased risk for poor health outcomes be educated and empowered to take action to reduce their risk. Further work is needed to improve effective patient communication and motivation strategies within a health care system steeped in a long-standing history of institutionalized racism and communication challenges.

SUMMARY

The social and economic effects of health disparities have an impact on the entire United States, if not global, population. Although the etiologies and manifestations of health care disparities are complex, with contributors at the patient, provider, and systems levels, important advances are being made and there is reason to be hopeful for significant strides in the future. Obstetrician-gynecologists have the unique opportunity to aid in the elimination of racial and ethnic disparities that affect not only the women they directly serve but also their children and future generations of their families.

Health and health care are fundamental to the well-being, productivity, and viability of communities. Inequities in health outcomes and care, therefore, pose real threats to the nation's well-being. Continuing the progress toward ending racial and ethnic disparities and ensuring health equity will take contributions and investment from participants at all levels of the health care system.

REFERENCES

1. Braveman P. Health disparities and health equity: concepts and measurement. Annu Rev Public Health 2006;27:167–94.
2. Jorde LB, Wooding SP. Genetic variation, classification and 'race'. Nat Genet 2004;36:S28–33.
3. National Center for Health Statistics. Resident population, by age, sex and Hispanic origins: United States, selected years 1950-2013. In: Health, United States, 2014: with special feature on adults aged 55–64. Hyattsvill (MD): NCHS; 2015. p. 55. Available at: http://www.cdc.gov/nchs/data/hus/2014/001.pdf. Accessed July 10, 2016.
4. Annual Estimates of the Resident Population by Sex, Race Alone or in Combination, and Hispanic Origin for the United States, States and Counties: April 1, 2010 to July 1, 2015. 2015 Population Estimates. In: United States Census Bureau, American Fact Finder. Available at: http://factfinder.census.gov/faces/tableservi ces/jsf/pages/productview.xhtml?src=bkmk. Accessed July 9, 2016.
5. Ayanian JZ. The costs of racial disparities in health care. Harvard Business Review 2015.
6. Owen CM, Goldstein EH, Clayton JA, et al. Racial and ethnic health disparities in reproductive medicine: an evidence-based overview. Semin Reprod Med 2013; 31:317–24.
7. Grobman WA, Bailit JL, Rice MM, et al. Racial and ethnic disparities in maternal morbidity and obstetric care. Obstet Gynecol 2015;125:1460–7.
8. Bryant A, Worjoloh A, Caughey A, et al. Racial/ethnic disparities in obstetrical outcomes and care: prevalence and determinants. Am J Obstet Gynecol 2010;202: 335–43.
9. Bryant AS, Washington S, Kuppermann M, et al. Quality and equality in obstetric care: racial and ethnic differences in caesarean section delivery rates. Paediatr Perinat Epidemiol 2009;23:454–62.
10. Borrero S, Moore CG, Qin L, et al. Unintended pregnancy influences racial disparity in tubal sterilization rates. J Gen Intern Med 2010;25:122–8.
11. Hoover KW, Parsell BW, Leichliter JS, et al. Continuing need for sexually transmitted disease clinics after the affordable care act. Am J Public Health 2015; 105(Suppl 5):S690–5.
12. Institute of Medicine. Unequal treatment: confronting racial and ethnic disparities in health care. Washington, DC: National Academics Press; 2003.
13. ACOG Committee on Obstetrics. ACOG Practice Bulletin No. 78: hemoglobinopathies in pregnancy. Obstet Gynecol 2007;109:229–37.
14. American College of Obstetricians and Gynecologists Committee on Genetics. ACOG Committee Opinion No. 486: update on carrier screening for cystic fibrosis. Obstet Gynecol 2011;117:1028–31.
15. Gamble VN. Under the shadow of Tuskegee: African Americans and health care. Am J Public Health 1997;87:1773–8.
16. Stern AM. Sterilized in the name of public health: race, immigration, and reproductive control in modern California. Am J Public Health 2005;95:1128–38.
17. Jacobs EA, Rolle I, Ferrans CE, et al. Understanding African Americans' views of the trustworthiness of physicians. J Gen Intern Med 2006;21:642–7.
18. Lind JN, Perrine CG, Li R, et al. Racial disparities in access to maternity care practices that support breastfeeding - United States, 2011. MMWR Morb Mortal Wkly Rep 2014;63:725–8.
19. Street DJ, Lewallen LP. The influence of culture on breast-feeding decisions by African American and white women. J Perinat Neonatal Nurs 2013;27:43–51.

20. Lundquist J, Xu Z, Barfield W, et al. Do black-white racial disparities in breast-feeding persist in the military community? Matern Child Health J 2015;19:419–27.

21. McGinnis JM, Foege WH. Actual causes of death in the United States. JAMA 1993;270:2207–12.

22. Thornton CM, Conway TL, Cain KL, et al. Disparities in Pedestrian streetscape environments by income and race/ethnicity. SSM Popul Health 2016;2:206–16.

23. Brown SD, Ehrlich SF, Kubo A, et al. Lifestyle behaviors and ethnic identity among diverse women at high risk for type 2 diabetes. Soc Sci Med 2016;160:87–93.

24. Haughton CF, Wang ML, Lemon SC. Racial/ethnic disparities in meeting 5-2-1-0 recommendations among children and adolescents in the United States. J Pediatr 2016;175:188–94.e1.

25. Borders AE, Wolfe K, Qadir S, et al. Racial/ethnic differences in self-reported and biologic measures of chronic stress in pregnancy. J Perinatol 2015;35:580–4.

26. A Sampling of Jim Crow laws. In: Learn NC. Available at: http://www.learnnc.org/lp/editions/nchist-newcentury/5103. Accessed July 9, 2016.

27. Chapman EN, Kaatz A, Carnes M. Physicians and implicit bias: how doctors may unwittingly perpetuate health care disparities. J Gen Intern Med 2013;28:1504–10.

28. Heins JK, Heins A, Grammas M, et al. Disparities in analgesia and opioid pre-scribing practices for patients with musculoskeletal pain in the emergency department. J Emerg Nurs 2006;32:219–24.

29. Miner J, Biros MH, Trainor A, et al. Patient and physician perceptions as risk factors for oligoanalgesia: a prospective observational study of the relief of pain in the emergency department. Acad Emerg Med 2006;13:140–6.

30. Todd KH, Lee T, Hoffman JR. The effect of ethnicity on physician estimates of pain severity in patients with isolated extremity trauma. JAMA 1994;271:925–8.

31. Hoffman KM, Trawalter S, Axt JR, et al. Racial bias in pain assessment and treatment recommendations, and false beliefs about biological differences between blacks and whites. Proc Natl Acad Sci U S A 2016;113:4296–301.

32. Canto JG, Allison JJ, Kiefe CI, et al. Relation of race and sex to the use of reperfusion therapy in Medicare beneficiaries with acute myocardial infarction. N Engl J Med 2000;342:1094–100.

33. Taylor HA Jr, Canto JG, Sanderson B, et al. Management and outcomes for black patients with acute myocardial infarction in the reperfusion era. National Registry of Myocardial Infarction 2 Investigators. Am J Cardiol 1998;82:1019–23.

34. Greenwald AG, Poehlman TA, Uhlmann EL, et al. Understanding and using the implicit association test: III. Meta-analysis of predictive validity. J Pers Soc Psychol 2009;97:17–41.

35. Green AR, Carney DR, Pallin DJ, et al. Implicit bias among physicians and its prediction of thrombolysis decisions for black and white patients. J Gen Intern Med 2007;22:1231–8.

36. Association of American Medical Colleges. What You Don't Know: The Science of Unconscious Bias and What to Do About It in the Search and Recruitment Process. Available at: https://www.aamc.org/initiatives/leadership/recruitment/178420/unconscious_bias.html. Accessed July 9, 2016.

37. Spettel S, White MD. The portrayal of J. Marion Sims' controversial surgical legacy. J Urol 2011;185:2424–7.

38. Gambino M. Fevered decisions: race, ethics, and clinical vulnerability in the malarial treatment of neurosyphilis, 1922-1953. Hastings Cent Rep 2015;45:39–50.

39. Kohler BA, Sherman RL, Howlader N, et al. Annual report to the nation on the status of cancer, 1975-2011, featuring incidence of breast cancer subtypes by race/ethnicity, poverty, and state. J Natl Cancer Inst 2015;107:djv048.
40. Centers for Disease Control and Prevention (CDC). Human papillomavirus-associated cancers - United States, 2004-2008. MMWR Morb Mortal Wkly Rep 2012;61:258–61.
41. Martinez G, Chandra A, Febo-Vazquez I, et al. Use of family planning and related medical services among women aged 15-44 in the United States: National Survey of Family Growth, 2006-2010. Natl Health Stat Report 2013;(68):1–16, 20.
42. Henley SJ, Singh SD, King J, et al. Invasive cancer incidence and survival–United States, 2011. MMWR Morb Mortal Wkly Rep 2015;64:237–42.
43. National Healthcare Quality and Disparities Report and 5th Anniversary Update on the National Quality Strategy. 2015. Available at: http://www.ahrq.gov/sites/default/files/wysiwyg/research/findings/nhqrdr/nhqdr15/2015nhqdr.pdf. Accessed July 10, 2016.
44. Burchard EG, Oh SS, Foreman MG, et al. Moving toward true inclusion of racial/ethnic minorities in federally funded studies. A key step for achieving respiratory health equality in the United States. Am J Respir Crit Care Med 2015;191:514–21.
45. Wendler D, Kington R, Madans J, et al. Are racial and ethnic minorities less willing to participate in health research? PLoS Med 2006;3:e19.
46. Racial and Ethnic Categories and Definition for NIH Diversity Programs and for Other Reporting Purposes. Issued by National Institutes of Health (NIH) on April 8, 2015. Available at: http://grants.nih.gov/grants/guide/notice-files/NOT-OD-15-089.html. Accessed July 11, 2016.
47. Tanaka M, Jaamaa G, Kaiser M, et al. Racial disparity in hypertensive disorders of pregnancy in New York State: a 10-year longitudinal population-based study. Am J Public Health 2007;97:163–70.
48. Velez Edwards DR, Hartmann KE. Racial differences in risk of spontaneous abortions associated with periconceptional over-the-counter nonsteroidal anti-inflammatory drug exposure. Ann Epidemiol 2014;24:111–5.e1.
49. Nguyen TT, Kaufman JS, Whitsel EA, et al. Racial differences in blood pressure response to calcium channel blocker monotherapy: a meta-analysis. Am J Hypertens 2009;22:911–7.
50. The American College of Obstetrics and Gynecologists Committee Opinion Number 649. Racial and Ethnic Disparities in Obstetrics and Gynecology. December 2015.
51. Eliminating Racial/Ethnic Disparities in Health Care: What are the Options? Available at: http://kff.org/disparities-policy/issue-brief/eliminating-racialethnic-disparities-in-health-care-what/#back9. Accessed July 9, 2016.
52. Racial and Ethnic Categories and Definitions for NIH Diversity Programs and for Other Reporting Purposes. April 8, 2015. Available at: http://grants.nih.gov/grants/guide/notice-files/NOT-OD-15-089.html. Accessed July 11, 2016.
53. Diversity in the Physician Workforce: Facts & Figures 2014. Section II: Current Status of the U.S. Physician Workforce. Available at: http://aamcdiversityfactsandfigures.org/section-ii-current-status-of-us-physician-workforce/. Accessed July 10, 2016.
54. American Association of Colleges of Nursing. Fact Sheet: Enhancing Diversity in the Nursing Workforce. Available at: http://www.aacn.nche.edu/media-relations/diversityFS.pdf. Accessed July 12, 2016.
55. Kurek K, Teevan BE, Zlateva I, et al. Patient-provider social concordance and health outcomes in patients with type 2 diabetes: a retrospective study from a

large federally qualified health center in Connecticut. J Racial Ethn Health Disparities 2016;3:217–24.

56. Meghani SH, Brooks JM, Gipson-Jones T, et al. Patient-provider race-concordance: does it matter in improving minority patients' health outcomes? Ethn Health 2009;14:107–30.

57. Saha S, Komaromy M, Koepsell TD, et al. Patient-physician racial concordance and the perceived quality and use of health care. Arch Intern Med 1999;159: 997–1004.

58. Laveist TA, Nuru-Jeter A. Is doctor-patient race concordance associated with greater satisfaction with care? J Health Soc Behav 2002;43:296–306.

59. Jackson CS, Gracia JN. Addressing health and health-care disparities: the role of a diverse workforce and the social determinants of health. Public Health Rep 2014;129(Suppl 2):57–61.

60. Narayan MC. The national standards for culturally and linguistically appropriate services in health care. Care Manag J 2001;3:77–83.

51.

Quality of Care and Disparities in Obstetrics

Elizabeth A. Howell, MD, MPP[a,b,*], Jennifer Zeitlin, DSc, MA[a,c]

KEYWORDS

- Disparities • Equity • Quality of care • Obstetrics • Quality improvement

KEY POINTS

- Quality of care in obstetrics varies widely and racial and ethnic disparities in obstetric and perinatal outcomes persist.
- Growing evidence suggests that quality of care contributes to racial and ethnic disparities in obstetric and perinatal outcomes.
- Quality measures should be used to track and reduce racial/ethnic disparities in obstetrics.

INTRODUCTION

Four million births occur annually in the United States and childbirth is a leading reason for hospitalization.[1] Childbirth is the largest category for hospital admissions for commercial payers and Medicaid programs and the estimated annual hospital costs associated with childbirth and newborns are more than $100 billion.[2,3] The United States spends more on maternity care than any other country in the world, yet the US maternal mortality and infant mortality rates are among the highest of all industrialized countries.[4,5] Hospital quality is associated with obstetric and neonatal outcomes and

Supported by the National Institute on Minority Health and Health Disparities (R01MD007651) and by the Eunice Kennedy Shriver National Institute of Child Health and Human Development of the National Institutes of Health (R01HD078565). The content is solely the responsibility of the authors and does not necessarily represent the official views of the National Institutes of Health.

Disclosure Statement: The authors have nothing to disclose.

[a] Department of Population Health Science and Policy, Icahn School of Medicine at Mount Sinai, One Gustave L. Levy Place, New York, NY 10029, USA; [b] Department of Obstetrics, Gynecology, and Reproductive Science, Icahn School of Medicine at Mount Sinai, One Gustave L. Levy Place, New York, NY 10029, USA; [c] Inserm UMR 1153, Obstetrical, Perinatal and Pediatric Epidemiology Research Team (Epopé), Center for Epidemiology and Biostatistics Sorbonne Paris Cité, DHU Risks in Pregnancy, Paris Descartes University, Maternité Port Royal, 53 avenue de l'Observatoire, Paris 75014, France

* Corresponding author. Icahn School of Medicine at Mount Sinai, Box 1077, One Gustave L. Levy Place, New York, NY 10029.

E-mail address: elizabeth.howell@mountsinai.org

Obstet Gynecol Clin N Am 44 (2017) 13–25
http://dx.doi.org/10.1016/j.ogc.2016.10.002
0889-8545/17/© 2016 Elsevier Inc. All rights reserved.

growing attention is being paid to obstetric quality and safety as patients and payers are pressing the health care system to measure and improve quality of care.

At the same time there is a growing recognition of the intractable racial and ethnic disparities prevalent in obstetric and perinatal outcomes.[6] Persistent racial and ethnic disparities in maternal and infant outcomes exist between white women and minority women.[7,8] Infant mortality rates are twice as high and maternal mortality rates are 3 to 4 times higher in black women versus white women.[7,9] Infant and maternal mortality rates are also higher in some Hispanic and other minority groups compared with white women. The obstetrics literature has documented racial and ethnic disparities across a range of obstetric and perinatal outcomes.[10] Although there is a vast literature base documenting the association of social determinants of health (eg, poverty, lack of education, poor nutritional status, smoking, and neighborhoods) with adverse maternal and perinatal outcomes,[11] for the most part these factors are not modifiable solely by the health care system. Hospital quality is one of few modifiable factors that the health care system can address, yet few obstetric studies have linked quality of care with racial and ethnic disparities.

Data suggest that obstetric quality varies widely across US hospitals.[12,13] Complications associated with childbirth occur in up to one-quarter of deliveries and rates for these complications vary widely across hospitals.[14,15] Studies by Maternal-Fetal Medicine Units Network investigators have documented variation among the 25 hospitals in their network in postpartum hemorrhage (from 1% to 5%), peripartum infection (2%–10%), and severe perineal laceration among forceps deliveries (8%–48%).[15] One in 10 term infants experiences a neonatal complication, such as hypoxia, shock, or birth injury, and investigators have found that these rates vary 7-fold across hospitals.[16,17] Obstetric processes of care, such as use of oxytocin, episiotomy, and general anesthesia, have also been shown to vary widely across hospitals.[18] Studies have found 10-fold variation in cesarean delivery rates across hospitals.[19] In addition, variations in outcomes are related to structural measures of quality, such as personnel training and level of care. For instance, maternal complication rates are associated with obstetricians' residency programs and provider volume.[12,20]

The wide variation in obstetric outcomes across hospitals, poor overall performance on perinatal indicators, and persistent racial and ethnic disparities in obstetric and perinatal outcomes require innovative remedies that tackle these challenges together. Equity is 1 of the 6 essential domains of quality according to the Institute of Medicine yet little attention in obstetrics has focused on the intersection between quality of care and disparities.[21] A growing portfolio of perinatal quality metrics has been endorsed by governmental agencies and professional bodies and the Centers for Medicaid & Medicare Services now requires hospitals to report on a few of these metrics.[22] Whether these metrics measure dimensions of care relevant to racial/ethnic disparities is, however, unknown.

This article reviews the definitions of quality of care, health disparities, and health equity as they relate to obstetric care and outcomes. Current efforts and challenges in obstetric quality measurement are described and then studies documenting racial and ethnic disparities in outcomes and quality by the authors and other investigators are discussed. Three strategies that may help reduce racial and ethnic disparities by focusing on quality of care are suggested.

QUALITY OF CARE
Definition

The Institute of Medicine defines health care quality as "the degree to which health services for individuals and populations increase the likelihood of desired health outcomes and care consistent with current professional knowledge."[23] In its 2001 report, *Crossing the Quality Chasm*, the Institute of Medicine[21] called for a redesign of the US health care system and provided a framework for improvement through 6 dimensions of care. The aims were built around the core need for health care to be safe, effective, patient-centered, timely, efficient, and equitable. To achieve the goal of quality improvement and to track progress require a concerted effort to measure performance. Therefore, over the past decade a great deal of effort has gone into developing and using quality measures in an effort to improve quality. Many government agencies and professional bodies have developed quality measures with the goal of improving care, by detecting suboptimal care based on the traditional Donabedian model,[24] which assesses structure, process, and outcomes. Structural measures are generally applied to characteristics of the provider of care, including hospitals (eg, bed size), physicians (eg, board certification), or systems of care (eg, presence of electronic health records). Process measures focus on delivery of specific interventions and services to improve quality of care, such as medications or procedures. Outcome measures provide information on health outcomes, such as mortality, morbidity, and patient experience and satisfaction.

A 3-part classification of quality problems, which has been widely used since its inception in the early 1990s, focuses on overuse, underuse, and misuse.[25] Overuse is the provision of health services when their risks outweigh their benefits for the recipient of that care (eg, doing surgery on a patient who is not going to benefit from the procedure). Underuse is failure to provide a health service when their benefits exceed their risks (eg, immunizations). Misuse is the failure to effectively deliver a proved benefit so that its full potential benefit is not conveyed to the patient (eg, antibiotics in the setting of a cold).

HEALTH DISPARITIES AND HEALTH EQUITY
Definition

There is a growing focus on reducing disparities and promoting health equity in health and health care, and the field of obstetrics is no exception. The American College of Obstetricians and Gynecologists and other professional societies have prioritized reducing health disparities and published committee opinions and consensus statements.[26] There has been ambiguity, however, in exactly what a health disparity is.[27,28] The National Institutes of Health defined health disparities as differences in the incidence, prevalence, mortality, and burden of disease and other adverse health conditions that exist among specific population groups in the United States."[29] Disparities imply inequity or an injustice, however, rather than a simple difference.[30] The hallmark Institute of Medicine 2003 report on disparities, *Unequal Treatment*, defined disparities as "racial or ethnic differences in the quality of health-care that are not due to access-related factors or clinical needs, preferences, and appropriateness of intervention."[31]

Experts in the field have emphasized the importance of clarity about the concepts of health disparities and health equity and stressed the underlying notion of social justice.[28] Many rely on the originally conceived definition of a health disparity by The World Health Organization, "differences in health which are not only unnecessary and avoidable but, in addition, are considered unfair and unjust."[32] A recent government definition, Healthy People 2020, has included the concept of social justice in its definition of a health disparity: "... a particular type of health difference that is, closely linked with economic, social, or environmental disadvantage. Health disparities adversely affect groups of people who have systematically experienced greater social or economic obstacles to health based on their racial or ethnic group, religion, socioeconomic-status, gender, age, or mental health; cognitive, sensory, or physical disability; sexual orientation of gender identify, geographic location; or other characteristics historically linked to discrimination or exclusion."[28] A disparity is not simply a difference. Rather, it is a difference that has a systematic and negative impact on less advantaged groups.

A simple and helpful definition was given by Dr Paula Braveman: "Health equity and health disparities are intertwined. Health equity means social justice in health (ie, no one is denied the possibility to be healthy for belonging to a group that has historically been economically/socially disadvantaged). Health disparities are the metric we use to measure progress toward achieving health equity."[28]

QUALITY MEASUREMENT IN OBSTETRICS

Measuring quality of care in obstetrics is complex: it involves assessing care for 2 separate individuals. Improving care requires reducing obstetric interventions that can harm infants and mothers (eg, delivery) and avoiding suboptimal care, such as underutilization of antenatal steroids, which can lead to neonatal complication.[17] Imperfect quality measures coupled with wide variation in performance are current challenges in the field.

In recent years, numerous quality indicators have been proposed for measurement of obstetric care in the United States.[33] Patients, insurers, and providers all have a vested interest in the easy availability of obstetric indicators. Many of the traditional obstetric indicators are poor markers of obstetric quality because they happen too infrequently, must be extensively risk adjusted, and have not been linked to specific processes of care that can be improved on. Use of risk-adjusted primary cesarean delivery rates have been used as a marker of quality but studies have shown that primary cesarean delivery rates that are either below or above predicted can be associated with poor neonatal outcomes, making the use of risk-adjusted primary cesarean delivery rates problematic to assess quality.[33] Perineal lacerations have been recommended as a quality indicator because they are easily tracked using coding data. Their use is not endorsed by the American College of Obstetricians and Gynecologists as quality indicators because they are not defined uniformly and are associated with nonmodifiable risk factors and reducing the use of operative vaginal delivery, in an effort to decrease severe perineal lacerations, likely would result in an increased rate of cesarean delivery.[34]

In addition to shortcomings with specific quality indicators, another challenge in the field is feasibility. To monitor quality across hospitals, data must be available in routine sources to construct valid, reliable, and case mix–adjusted indicators. According to the National Quality Forum and experts in the field, quality measures must be evidence based, important, acceptable (precisely defined, reliable, valid, discriminatory, and risk adjusted if necessary and have consistent evidence linking process to outcomes), feasible, and usable.[35]

Currently there are several recommended obstetric quality indicators. **Table 1** lists some examples. The Agency for Healthcare Research and Quality (AHRQ) has proposed a set of obstetrics-related quality indicators for their inpatient, safety, and prevention indicators.[36] The National Quality Forum has endorsed 14 measures,[37] and some of these measures are now used by The Joint Commission as perinatal quality measures.[38] Currently the Centers for Medicare & Medicaid Services mandates hospitals to report one of these measures, the elective delivery measure that includes nonmedically indicated deliveries associated with medical induction.[22] The focus on

		Structure/Process/	Quality Problem
Measure Endorser	**Indicator**	**Outcome**	**Addressed**
The Joint Commission/NQF	Elective delivery	Outcome	Overuse
The Joint Commission/NQF	Cesarean delivery rate for low-risk first births	Outcome	Overuse
NQF	Incidence episiotomy	Process	Overuse
AHRQ	Cesarean delivery rate	Outcome	Overuse
AHRQ	Primary cesarean delivery rate	Outcome	Overuse
AHRQ	Obstetric trauma – vaginal with instrument	Outcome	Overuse
AHRQ	Obstetric trauma – vaginal without instrument	Outcome	Overuse
AHRQ	Obstetric trauma – cesarean delivery	Outcome	Overuse
NQF	Prophylactic antibiotics at cesarean births	Process	Underuse
NQF	Appropriate DVT prophylaxis in women Undergoing cesarean delivery	Process	Underuse
NQF	Intrapartum antibiotic prophylaxis for group B streptococcus	Process	Underuse
NQF	Infants under 1500 g delivered at appropriate site	Process/Structure	Underuse
The Joint Commission/NQF	Antenatal steroids	Process	Underuse
The Joint Commission/NQF	Exclusive breast milk feeding	Outcome	Underuse

Table 1
Examples of current obstetric quality indicators by quality problem addressed

Abbreviations: AHRQ, Agency for Healthcare Research and Quality; DVT, deep vein thrombosis; NQF, National Quality Forum.
Data from Refs.[36–38]

quality in maternity care extends internationally. Investigators in Europe have used a modified Delphi approach with use of an international multidisciplinary panel to select a list of indicators that reflect the quality of obstetric care in maternity units.[39] All these efforts have enriched the debate about obstetric quality considerably and have moved the field of quality measurement forward.

Although some strides have been made in maternity quality improvement, it is unclear whether the current portfolio of obstetric quality indicators is comprehensive enough to drive major improvement in the field. The authors' recent work has focused on assessing if obstetric quality indicators are associated with maternal and neonatal morbidity.[17] Whether hospital performance on 2 of The Joint Commission perinatal quality measures, elective (nonmedically indicated) deliveries at greater than or equal to 37 weeks and less than 39 weeks of gestation and cesarean delivery performed in low-risk mothers, were associated with hospital performance on severe maternal and term neonatal morbidity were examined. Wide variation was found among hospitals for elective deliveries performed before 39 weeks and for cesarean deliveries performed in low-risk mothers. Severe maternal morbidity and neonatal morbidity at term rates varied, 5-fold and 7-fold, respectively. There were no correlations, however, between performance on the hospital quality indicators and hospital maternal morbidity and neonatal morbidity rates. The authors concluded that quality indicators may not be sufficiently comprehensive for guiding quality improvement in obstetric care.[17] Other investigators have also argued that the current repertoire of quality indicators are not comprehensive.[16]

DISPARITIES, OUTCOMES, AND QUALITY
Disparities in Obstetric and Perinatal Outcomes

Half of all US births are to racial/ethnic minority women,[40–42] and racial/ethnic minorities suffer a disproportionate number of maternal deaths as well as other adverse obstetric and perinatal outcomes. African American women are 3 to 4 times more likely to die from pregnancy-related causes than white women. This represents the largest disparity among all the conventional population perinatal health measures.[7] Maternal mortality is also elevated among Native Americans/Native Alaskans, Asians/Pacific Islanders, and for certain subgroups of Latino women, including Puerto Ricans.[43–45] Maternal mortality ratios have increased over the past 3 decades,[46,47] despite advances in diagnosis and acute critical care.[48] In New York City, the most recent data demonstrate that black or African American women are 12 times more likely than whites to suffer a pregnancy-related death.[49] The increase in the black-white maternal mortality disparity was attributed to a 45% decline in maternal mortality among white women in New York City.[49]

Several pregnancy complications and comorbidities associated with maternal death are more common among minorities than whites. Potentially fatal complications of pregnancy include hemorrhage, hypertensive disorders of pregnancy, and cardiomyopathy and black women suffer greater mortality from all of them.[50] A leading cause of death in Hispanic women after pregnancy in 1 study was hypertensive disease, placing them at a 3-fold increased risk of death due to this complication.[43] Minority women have been found to have both higher prevalence and higher case fatality rates for these disorders and for more common problems, such as diabetes. A national study published in 2007 that investigated pregnancy-related mortality among black women versus white women found that black women did not have significantly higher prevalence of 5 specific pregnancy complications but for all 5 conditions black women had a case-fatality rate 2.4 to 3.3 times higher than that of white women.[51]

Reviews of racial/ethnic disparities in outcomes and care have documented disparities across several other maternal and perinatal outcomes.[10] Black women and Hispanic women have higher rates of severe maternal morbidity as well as diabetes and obesity. Asian women and Hispanic women are at greater risk of developing gestational diabetes. Disparities also exist in the prevalence and severity of several other maternal complications, including HIV and asthma.[10]

The disparities in adverse perinatal outcomes are well documented for minority versus white women. Part of the reason that the United States does so poorly overall and compared with other countries with respect to perinatal outcomes is the persistent disparities in outcomes between white women and minority women. In 2013, the infant mortality rate was much higher for blacks (11.11 deaths per 1000 live births), American Indians or Alaska Natives (7.61 deaths per 1000 live births), and Puerto Ricans (5.93 deaths per 1000 live births) versus whites (5.06 deaths per 1000 live births).[9] Preterm birth is more common among black women and Puerto Rican women than white women (16.3%, 13.0%, and 10.2% of births, respectively).[9] It has been estimated that disparities in preterm births are responsible for a major portion of the black-white and Puerto Rican–white disparities in infant mortality rates.[9] Racial/ethnic disparities exist in the prevalence of preterm birth, fetal growth restriction, fetal demise, and congenital anomalies.[10]

Disparities and Quality

Significant racial/ethnic disparities in obstetric and perinatal outcomes have been evident for decades. Yet, little research has investigated the association between obstetric quality and racial/ethnic disparities in these outcomes. Studies from other areas in medicine and more recently in obstetrics suggest that minorities receive care in different and lower-quality hospitals than whites.[52–54] Using data from the Nationwide Inpatient Sample, the authors found that blacks deliver in a concentrated set of hospitals and these hospitals have higher risk-adjusted severe maternal morbidity rates for both white deliveries and black deliveries.[54] The authors ranked hospitals by their proportion of black deliveries into high black-serving (top 5%), medium black-serving (5% to 25% range), and low black-serving hospitals and analyzed the risks of severe maternal morbidity for black women and white women by hospital black-serving status after adjusting for patient characteristics, comorbidities, hospital characteristics, and within-hospital clustering. Severe maternal morbidity occurred more frequently among black women than white women (25.8 vs 11.8 per 1000 deliveries, respectively; $P<.001$) and after adjustment this differential declined but remained elevated (18.8 vs 13.3 per 1000 deliveries, respectively; $P<.001$). Women who delivered in high and medium black-serving hospitals had elevated rates of severe maternal morbidity rates compared with those in low black-serving hospitals in adjusted analyses (**Fig. 1**).[54]

In another study focused on New York City, after adjustment for patient case mix, the authors found 7-fold variation in severe maternal morbidity rates and white deliveries were more likely to be delivered in the low-morbidity hospitals: 65% of white deliveries versus 23% of black deliveries occurred in hospitals in the lowest tertile for morbidity.[55] The authors estimated that black-white differences in delivery location may contribute as much as 47.7% of the racial disparity in severe maternal morbidity rates in New York City.[55] In pediatrics, research by the authors' team and others has also found that black very-low-birth-weight babies are more likely to be delivered in higher risk-adjusted very-low-birth-weight neonatal mortality hospitals,[56,57] and studies in other areas of medicine have demonstrated similar findings.[53] Studies of acute myocardial infarction treatment have shown that black patients tend to receive

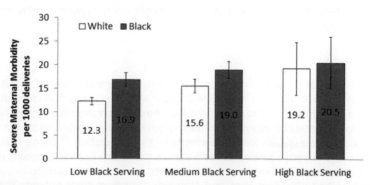

Fig. 1. Risk-adjusted severe maternal morbidity rates for black deliveries and white deliveries by site of care. (*From* Howell EA, Egorova N, Balbierz A, et al. Black-white differences in severe maternal morbidity and site of care. Am J Obstet Gynecol 2016;214(1):122.e5; with permission.)

care in hospitals with higher mortality rates and lower rates of effective evidence-based medical treatments compared with white patients.[52] Studies have demonstrated that blacks and whites receive care from different providers and the physicians treating black patients are less likely to be board certified and may have less access to important clinical resources than physicians treating white patients.[58]

Other investigators have also found differences in delivery-related indicators by hospital type and patients' race and ethnicity.[59] Investigators, using 7 state inpatient databases, investigated 15 delivery-related indicators (eg, obstetric trauma, would complications, complicated vaginal delivery, and hemorrhage) among white-serving, Hispanic-serving, and black-serving hospitals.[59] They found differences in delivery-related indicators by hospital type and overall lower performance of black-serving hospitals compared with white-serving and Hispanic-serving hospitals. The investigators concluded that obstetric quality measures are needed to track racial/ethnic disparities at the facility and populations levels.[59]

Disparities and Quality Indicators

Few obstetric quality measures have been used to track and reduce racial/ethnic disparities in obstetrics. The authors examined national trends and black-white differences in AHRQ obstetrics-related patient safety, inpatient quality indicators and inpatient neonatal and maternal mortality using national data,[60] including 3 Patient Safety Indicators—obstetric trauma (third-degree or fourth-degree laceration) with instrument, obstetric trauma without instrument, and birth trauma to neonate—and 4 Inpatient Quality Indicators—cesarean section rate, primary cesarean section rate, uncomplicated vaginal birth after cesarean section (VBAC), and all VBACs. All 3 patient safety indicators decreased over the 10-year study period and improvements occurred for both blacks and whites. For both blacks and whites, cesarean section rates increased by 60% to 65% and VBACs decreased by 70% to 75% over the study period. Despite improvements for blacks and whites, however, in some of these quality measures during the study period, the black-white maternal mortality gap widened and the neonatal mortality gap persisted. The authors concluded that AHRQ quality measures related to procedures do not contribute to understanding of persistent racial/ethnic disparities in maternal or neonatal inpatient mortality.[60]

Although the Centers for Disease Control and Prevention tracks several important population health measures by race and ethnicity (eg, maternal mortality, severe maternal morbidity, preterm birth, and infant mortality), few in the field of obstetrics track quality measures by race and ethnicity and establish targeted quality improvement efforts to reduce disparities.

DISCUSSION – NEXT STEPS

There is a need to develop, track, and improve on quality measures that are sensitive to disparities in obstetrics and there are 3 major steps suggested to move forward (**Fig. 2**). First, The Joint Commission and others have recommended stratifying quality information by race and ethnicity, as well as other sociodemographics, in an effort to track and improve quality for all segments of the population.[61] Disparities dashboards have been used in some hospitals across the nation to stratify quality metrics by race and ethnicity. The first step in this process is to ensure that hospitals and clinicians collect self-identified race and ethnicity data from their patients.[61] Proper training of staff is required and patient education is needed to explain why this information is important. Next, obstetric quality measures should be stratified by race and ethnicity and reviewed by leadership and staff. Quality gaps should be identified

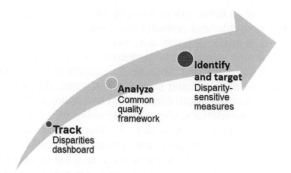

Fig. 2. Three strategies to reduce disparities by focusing on quality of care.

and targeted interventions should be introduced to reduce disparities.[61] Progress should be monitored.

Second, a great deal of research and progress can be made by using the common quality-of-care framework of overuse, underuse, and misuse in the setting of racial and ethnic disparities in obstetrics to better understand where to go from here.[25] Two current perinatal indicators of The Joint Commission, elective delivery before 39 weeks and low-risk cesarean, are both primarily overuse measures.[17,38] Overutilization of both of these measures may be associated with poor outcomes for babies and mothers but the authors' recent data indicate that neither is correlated with severe maternal morbidity or neonatal morbidity at term.[17] Data demonstrate that racial and ethnic disparities in severe maternal morbidity and neonatal morbidity at term exist.[17] Clearly, additional quality measures are needed that are patient centered and correlated with important obstetric outcomes, such as severe maternal morbidity and neonatal morbidity. Furthermore, data from other areas of medicine suggest that overuse of procedures may be more likely to occur in whites than nonwhites.[62] The extent to which overuse is a quality problem in obstetrics has been studied in 1 area, cesarean delivery. Several studies have documented higher risks of cesarean delivery among nonwhite women compared with white women even after adjusting for patient factors.[63] The extent to which overuse contributes to disparities in obstetric outcomes, however, has not been fully investigated. In contrast, the field of disparities is full of examples of underuse, underutilization of procedures, and treatments for minorities.[31] This has also been shown in the setting of obstetrics.[10]

Third, an expanded set of quality measures are needed in the field. The National Quality Forum in 2008 developed criteria for "disparities sensitive" measures.[64] The guiding principles were

1. How prevalent was the condition in the disparity population?
2. What is the impact of the condition for the health of the disparity population?
3. How strong is the evidence linking improvement in the measure to improved outcomes for any group but particularly for members of disparity populations?
4. How large is the disparity gap in quality?
5. Is the measure actionable?[64]

These guiding principles should be used to develop a robust set of quality measures that can help track and reduce disparities. Examples may be the use of antibiotics in the setting of preterm labor or the use of progesterone in specific high-risk groups for the prevention of preterm birth.

Approximately half of all births are to minority mothers, and persistent racial and ethnic disparities in obstetric and perinatal outcomes exist. Efforts to reduce racial and ethnic disparities in maternal health are needed. Although much of the focus on reducing racial and ethnic disparities in obstetrics examines social determinants of health, there is ample evidence that differences in quality of care contribute to racial and ethnic disparities in obstetric and perinatal outcomes. Quality of care is one of few modifiable factors that the health care system can address. This article proposes 3 steps in an effort to develop, track, and improve quality and reduce disparities in obstetrics. The use of disparities dashboards to monitor and intervene on racial/ethnic disparities in obstetric quality measures, the assessment of quality problems related to disparities using a common quality framework, and the development of disparities-sensitive metrics in the field of obstetrics can help reduce current quality gaps in the care provided to patients.

REFERENCES

1. DeFrances CJ, Cullen KA, Kozak LJ. National Hospital Discharge Survey: 2005 annual summary with detailed diagnosis and procedure data. Vital Health Stat 13 2007;(165):1–209.
2. Wier LM, Andrews RM. The National Hospital Bill: The Most Expensive Conditions by Payer, 2008. HCUP Statistical Brief #107. Rockville (MD): Agency for Healthcare Research and Quality; 2011. Available at: http://www.hcup-us.ahrq.gov/reports/statbriefs/sb107.pdf.
3. Transforming Maternity Care – United States Maternity Care Facts and Figures. 2012. Available at: http://transform.childbirthconnection.org/resources/datacenter/factsandfigures/. Accessed July 16, 2016.
4. MacDorman MF, Mathews TJ. Behind international rankings of infant mortality: how the United States compares with Europe. Int J Health Serv 2010;40(4):577–88.
5. Amnesty International. Deadly delivery: the maternal health care crisis in the US. London: Amnesty International; 2010.
6. Willis E, McManus P, Magallanes N, et al. Conquering racial disparities in perinatal outcomes. Clin Perinatol 2014;41(4):847–75.
7. Callaghan WM. Overview of maternal mortality in the United States. Semin Perinatol 2012;36(1):2–6.
8. Mathews TJ, MacDorman MF. Infant mortality statistics from the 2006 period linked birth/infant death data set. Natl Vital Stat Rep 2010;57(17):1–32.
9. Matthews TJ, MacDorman MF, Thoma ME. Infant mortality statistics from the 2013 period linked birth/infant death data set. Natl Vital Stat Rep 2015;64(9):1–30.
10. Bryant AS, Worjoloh A, Caughey AB, et al. Racial/ethnic disparities in obstetric outcomes and care: prevalence and determinants. Am J Obstet Gynecol 2010; 202(4):335–43.
11. Institute of Medicine. Preterm births: causes, consequences and prevention. Washington, DC: The National Academy of Science; 2006.
12. Asch DA, Nicholson S, Srinivas S, et al. Evaluating obstetrical residency programs using patient outcomes. JAMA 2009;302(12):1277–83.
13. Glance LG, Dick AW, Glantz JC, et al. Rates of major obstetrical complications vary almost fivefold among US hospitals. Health Aff (Millwood) 2014;33(8):1330–6.
14. Gregory KD, Fridman M, Shah S, et al. Global measures of quality- and patient safety-related childbirth outcomes: should we monitor adverse or ideal rates? Am J Obstet Gynecol 2009;200(6):681.e1-7.

15. Bailit JL, Grobman WA, Rice MM, et al. Risk-adjusted models for adverse obstetric outcomes and variation in risk-adjusted outcomes across hospitals. Am J Obstet Gynecol 2013;209(5):446.e1-30.
16. Korst LM, Fridman M, Michael CL, et al. Monitoring childbirth morbidity using hospital discharge data: further development and application of a composite measure. Am J Obstet Gynecol 2014;211(3):268.e1-16.
17. Howell EA, Zeitlin J, Hebert PL, et al. Association between hospital-level obstetric quality indicators and maternal and neonatal morbidity. JAMA 2014;312(15): 1531-41.
18. Grobman WA, Bailit JL, Rice MM, et al. Can differences in obstetric outcomes be explained by differences in the care provided? The MFMU Network APEX Study. Am J Obstet Gynecol 2014;211(2):147.e1-16.
19. Kozhimannil KB, Law MR, Virnig BA. Cesarean delivery rates vary tenfold among US hospitals; reducing variation may address quality and cost issues. Health Aff (Millwood) 2013;32(3):527-35.
20. Janakiraman V, Lazar J, Joynt KE, et al. Hospital volume, provider volume, and complications after childbirth in U.S. hospitals. Obstet Gynecol 2011;118(3): 521-7.
21. Institute of Medicine (IOM). Crossing the quality chasm: a new health system for the 21st century. Washington, DC: National Academy Press; 2001.
22. Center for Medicare and Medicaid Services. Hospital compare. Available at: http://www.cms.gov/Medicare/Quality-Initiatives-Patient-Assessment-Instruments/HospitalQualityInits/HospitalCompare.html. Accessed July 16, 2016.
23. Lohr K, Committee to Design a Strategy for Quality Review and Assurance in Medicare, editors. Medicare: a strategy for quality assurance, vol. 1. Washington, DC: IOM, National Academy Press; 1990.
24. Boulkedid R, Alberti C, Sibony O. Quality indicator development and implementation in maternity units. Best Pract Res Clin Obstet Gynaecol 2013;27(4): 609-19.
25. Chassin MR. Quality of care. Time to act. JAMA 1991;266(24):3472-3.
26. ACOG Committee Opinion No. 649: racial and ethnic disparities in obstetrics and gynecology. Obstet Gynecol 2015;126(6):e130-4.
27. Dehlendorf C, Bryant AS, Huddleston HG, et al. Health disparities: definitions and measurements. Am J Obstet Gynecol 2010;202(3):212-3.
28. Braveman P. What are health disparities and health equity? We need to be clear. Public Health Rep 2014;129(Suppl 2):5-8.
29. Braveman PA, Kumanyika S, Fielding J, et al. Health disparities and health equity: the issue is justice. Am J Public Health 2011;101(Suppl 1):S149-55.
30. Hebert PL, Sisk JE, Howell EA. When does a difference become a disparity? Conceptualizing racial and ethnic disparities in health. Health Aff (Millwood) 2008;27(2):374-82.
31. Smedley BD, Stith AY, Nelson AR, editors. Unequal treatment: confronting racial and ethnic disparities in health care. Washington, DC: National Academies Press; 2003.
32. Whitehead M. The concepts and principles of equity and health. Health Promot Int 1991;6(3):217-28.
33. Bailit JL. Measuring the quality of inpatient obstetrical care. Obstet Gynecol Surv 2007;62(3):207-13.
34. Committee on Obstetric Practice. ACOG Committee Opinion No. 647: limitations of Perineal Lacerations as an Obstetric Quality Measure. Obstet Gynecol 2015; 126(5):e108-11.

35. Main EK. New perinatal quality measures from the National Quality Forum, the Joint Commission and the Leapfrog Group. Curr Opin Obstet Gynecol 2009; 21(6):532–40.

36. Agency for Healthcare Research and Quality. AHRQ quality indicators. Available at: http://www.qualityindicators.ahrq.gov/. Accessed July 16, 2016.

37. National Quality Forum. NQF endorses perinatal measures. 2012. Available at: http://www.qualityforum.org/News_And_Resources/Press_Releases/2012/NQF_Endorses_Perinatal_Measures.aspx. Accessed July 16, 2016.

38. The Joint Commission. Specifications Manual for Joint Commission National Quality Measures (v2016A). 2016. Available at: https://manual.jointcommission.org/releases/TJC2016A/. Accessed July 16, 2016.

39. Boulkedid R, Sibony O, Goffinet F, et al. Quality indicators for continuous monitoring to improve maternal and infant health in maternity departments: a modified Delphi survey of an international multidisciplinary panel. PLoS One 2013;8(4): e60663.

40. Martin JA, Hamilton BE, Sutton PD, et al. Births: final data for 2005. Natl Vital Stat Rep 2007;56(6):1–103.

41. Martin JA, Hamilton BE, Sutton PD, et al. Births: final data for 2004. Natl Vital Stat Rep 2006;55(1):1–101.

42. Tavernise S. Whites account for under half of Births in U.S. - NYTimes.com. The New Yorks Times 2012. Available at: http://www.nytimes.com/2012/05/17/us/whites-account-for-under-half-of-births-in-us.html?pagewanted=2&_r=1&ref=race. Accessed May 17, 2012.

43. Hopkins FW, MacKay AP, Koonin LM, et al. Pregnancy-related mortality in Hispanic women in the United States. Obstet Gynecol 1999;94(5 Pt 1):747–52.

44. CDC. Pregnancy-related deaths among Hispanic, Asian/Pacific Islander, and American Indian/Alaska Native women–United States, 1991-1997. MMWR Morb Mortal Wkly Rep 2001;50(18):361–4.

45. Gray KE, Wallace ER, Nelson KR, et al. Population-based study of risk factors for severe maternal morbidity. Paediatr Perinat Epidemiol 2012;26(6):506–14.

46. Berg CJ, Atrash HK, Koonin LM, et al. Pregnancy-related mortality in the United States, 1987-1990. Obstet Gynecol 1996;88(2):161–7.

47. Heron M, Hoyert DL, Murphy SL, et al. Deaths: final data for 2006. Natl Vital Stat Rep 2009;57(14):1–134.

48. Pahlavan P, Nezhat C. Hemorrhage in obstetrics and gynecology. Curr Opin Obstet Gynecol 2001;13(4):419–24.

49. New York City Department of Health and Mental Hygiene Bureau of Maternal Health. Pregnancy-Associated Mortality New York City, 2006-2010. The NYC Department of Mental Health and Hygiene: New York. 2015.

50. Harper MA, Espeland MA, Dugan E, et al. Racial disparity in pregnancy-related mortality following a live birth outcome. Ann Epidemiol 2004;14(4):274–9.

51. Tucker MJ, Berg CJ, Callaghan WM, et al. The Black–White Disparity in Pregnancy-Related Mortality from 5 Conditions: Differences in Prevalence and Case-Fatality Rates. Am J Public Health 2007;97(2):247–51.

52. Barnato AE, Lucas FL, Staiger D, et al. Hospital-level racial disparities in acute myocardial infarction treatment and outcomes. Med Care 2005;43(4):308–19.

53. Cheng EM, Keyhani S, Ofner S, et al. Lower use of carotid artery imaging at minority-serving hospitals. Neurology 2012;79(2):138–44.

54. Howell EA, Egorova N, Balbierz A, et al. Black-white differences in severe maternal morbidity and site of care. Am J Obstet Gynecol 2016;214(1):122.e1-7.

55. Howell EA, Egorova NN, Balbierz A, et al. Site of delivery contribution to black-white severe maternal morbidity disparity. Am J Obstet Gynecol 2016;215(2): 143–52.
56. Howell EA, Hebert P, Chatterjee S, et al. Black/white differences in very low birth weight neonatal mortality rates among New York City hospitals. Pediatrics 2008; 121(3):e407–15.
57. Morales LS, Staiger D, Horbar JD, et al. Mortality among very low-birthweight infants in hospitals serving minority populations. Am J Public Health 2005;95(12): 2206–12.
58. Bach PB, Pham HH, Schrag D, et al. Primary care physicians who treat blacks and whites. N Engl J Med 2004;351(6):575–84.
59. Creanga AA, Bateman BT, Mhyre JM, et al. Performance of racial and ethnic minority-serving hospitals on delivery-related indicators. Am J Obstet Gynecol 2014;211(6):647.e1-16.
60. Howell EA, Zeitlin J, Hebert P, et al. Paradoxical trends and racial differences in obstetric quality and neonatal and maternal mortality. Obstet Gynecol 2013; 121(6):1201–8.
61. Ramos R, Davis JL, Ross T, et al. Measuring health disparities and health inequities: do you have REGAL data? Qual Manag Health Care 2012;21(3):176–87.
62. Kressin NR, Groeneveld PW. Race/Ethnicity and overuse of care: a systematic review. Milbank Q 2015;93(1):112–38.
63. Bryant AS, Washington S, Kuppermann M, et al. Quality and equality in obstetric care: racial and ethnic differences in caesarean section delivery rates. Paediatr Perinat Epidemiol 2009;23(5):454–62.
64. National Quality Forum. National Voluntary Consensus Standards for Ambulatory Care — Measuring Healthcare Disparities. 2008. Available at: http://www.quality forum.org/Publications/2008/03/National_Voluntary_Consensus_Standards_for_Ambulatory_Care%e2%80%94Measuring_Healthcare_Disparities.aspx. Accessed July 16, 2016.

Reassessing Unintended Pregnancy

Toward a Patient-centered Approach to Family Planning

Jessica E. Morse, MD, MPH[a],*, Shanthi Ramesh, MD[a],
Andrea Jackson, MD, MAS[b]

KEYWORDS

- Underserved women • Unintended pregnancy • Patient-centered care
- Family planning • Reproductive life planning • Contraceptive counseling
- Disparities

KEY POINTS

- Underserved women, particularly those who are low income and of racial and ethnic minorities, experience a disproportionate share of unintended pregnancies in the United States.
- Unintended pregnancy rates are general markers of women's health and status but may not accurately capture women's experiences of these pregnancies.
- A patient-centered approach to family planning optimizes women's reproductive preferences and is cognizant of historical harms and current disparities.
- Clinicians, researchers, and policy makers can all adopt a patient-centered approach to help underserved women regain their reproductive autonomy.

INTRODUCTION

Low-income women and racial and ethnic minorities experience a disproportionate share of unintended pregnancies in the United States.[1] Although unintended pregnancy rates are general markers of women's health and status, they may not accurately capture women's experiences of these pregnancies or their social circumstances. The authors suggest a patient-centered approach to family planning that

Disclosure: The authors have nothing to disclose.
[a] Family Planning Division, Department of Obstetrics & Gynecology, University of North Carolina, 101 Manning Drive, Campus Box #7570, Chapel Hill, NC 27514, USA; [b] Department of Obstetrics, Gynecology & Reproductive Sciences, University of California, 2356 Sutter Street, 5th Floor, San Francisco, CA 94143, USA
* Corresponding author.
E-mail address: Jessica_morse@med.unc.edu

Obstet Gynecol Clin N Am 44 (2017) 27–40
http://dx.doi.org/10.1016/j.ogc.2016.10.003
0889-8545/17/© 2016 Elsevier Inc. All rights reserved.

optimizes women's reproductive preferences and is cognizant of historical harms and current disparities. Such an approach addresses the issue of unintended pregnancy in a comprehensive and nuanced way that places the women's preferences at the center of the contraceptive decision-making process, research, and public health policies. Clinicians, researchers, and policy makers can all adopt a patient-centered approach to help underserved women regain their reproductive autonomy.

REASSESSING UNINTENDED PREGNANCY
What Is Unintended Pregnancy?

In the United States and abroad, unintended pregnancy rates are considered a key indicator of women's autonomy and control over their reproductive lives and are used extensively in research, policy, and program planning. Since the introduction of this metric as a marker for reproductive health in the 1940s, numerous political, economic, and cultural changes have taken place that have a profound impact on how people perceive sexuality, fertility, and even medical care. Some of these changes may suggest that it is time to reassess what is being measured when unintended pregnancy is measured.

An unintended pregnancy was traditionally defined as a pregnancy that, at the time of conception, was either mistimed (the mother wanted the pregnancy to occur at a later time) or unwanted (the mother did not want it to occur at that time or any time in the future). By default, pregnancies that occur at the right time, later than desired, or to women who are indifferent about the pregnancy are considered intended.[2] Unintended pregnancy is a subjective metric that retrospectively asks a woman to describe her feelings about her pregnancy. Data are generally collected via survey, and, almost exclusively, from the woman. The National Survey of Family Growth (NSFG) and Pregnancy Risk Assessment Monitoring Survey (PRAMS), two commonly used tools for national-level data on unintended pregnancy, assess pregnancy intendedness by inquiring about pregnancy timing (too soon, too late, or just right). Other survey tools use questions about happiness relative to pregnancy, or consideration of pregnancy termination, suggesting that unintended pregnancy rates may vary based on how the questions are asked.

What Is the Utility of Measuring Unintended Pregnancy?

Unintended pregnancy has long been considered a significant public health problem and has been used as a key indicator of women's overall health status and access to reproductive health services. Poor pregnancy outcomes, such as late entry to prenatal care, alcohol and tobacco use, and low birth weight, have been associated with unintended pregnancy.[3,4] Long-term impacts include lower economic and educational gains.[3–5] Although these negative impacts of unintended pregnancy are of great concern, it remains unclear to what extent they can be disentangled from the associated complex social and economic factors that may be driving them. The women most likely to experience unintended pregnancies are from socially marginalized communities: poor women, less educated women, and racial and ethnic minority women. These women are also more likely to experience poor pregnancy outcomes (both immediate and long term), whether a pregnancy was planned or not.[6–8] They are also more likely to live in communities of disenfranchisement, where decades of discriminatory policies result in limited access to health care and economic instability. Thus, some of the long-term outcomes of unintended pregnancy are hard to separate from these circumstances. Regardless of the imperfect definition and unclear associations with poor outcomes, unintended pregnancy is currently the best metric to evaluate the reproductive health of a society and community.

Who Experiences Unintended Pregnancy?

According to nationally representative data collected through the NSFG, 45% of the 6.1 million pregnancies in the United States in 2011 were unintended. Although this is a marked decline from 54% in 2008, there were still 45 unintended pregnancies for every 1000 women and girls aged 15 to 44 years.[9]

Although these trends in declining unintended pregnancy rates are cause for optimism, poor women still have 5-fold higher unintended pregnancy rates than their wealthier counterparts (**Fig. 1**)[9] and the differential rates across racial and ethnic groups remain (**Fig. 2**). In 2011, the unintended pregnancy rate among white, non-Hispanic women was 33 per 1000 reproductive-aged women. It was more than twice as high among black non-Hispanic women (79 per 1000) and almost double among Hispanic women (58 per 1000).

CONCERNS ABOUT USING UNINTENDED PREGNANCY AS A MARKER IN A CLINICAL ENCOUNTER

Although the dichotomized question of whether or not a pregnancy was intended may be useful for examining the large-scale public health of a community, in an individual clinical encounter, this may not be the case. For many women, especially socially disenfranchised women, clearly defining pregnancy intentions before conception is not necessarily an active process.[10,11] This ambivalence or unclear intention is often reflected in contraceptive and sexual practices, and may explain (in part) how such a large proportion of women with unintended pregnancies report having recently used contraception.[12,13] Although ambivalence has been associated with less effective contraceptive use,[14,15] some qualitative work among low-income, urban white and black women showed that pregnancy intentions and contraceptive behavior are often not well matched.[10,11] The feelings driving these seemingly discrepant behaviors are reflected in the happiness women may describe about a pregnancy, even while calling

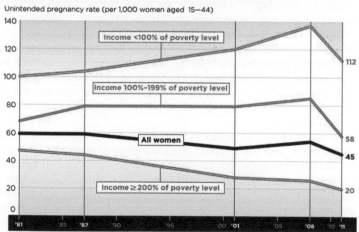

Large disparities by income remain

Unintended pregnancy rate (per 1,000 women aged 15—44)

Income <100% of poverty level — 112

Income 100%-199% of poverty level

All women — 58

Income ≥200% of poverty level — 45, 20

'81 '85 '87 '90 '95 '00 '01 '05 '08 '10 '11

Fig. 1. Unintended pregnancy rates by income (per 1000 women aged 15–44 years). The 2011 federal poverty level was $22,350 for a family of 4. (*From* Guttmacher Institute. The U.S. unintended pregnancy rate is at its lowest in 30 years, Infographic. New York: Guttmacher Institute; 2016. Available at: https://www.guttmacher.org/infographic/2016/us-unintended-pregnancy-rate-its-lowest-30-years; with permission.)

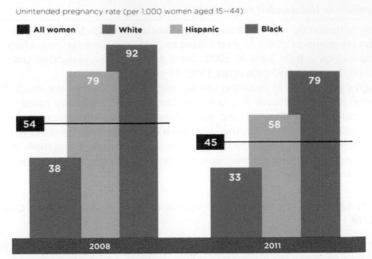

Unintended pregnancy rate (per 1,000 women aged 15–44)

■ All women   ■ White   ■ Hispanic   ■ Black

Fig. 2. Unintended pregnancy rates across racial and ethnic groups (per 1000 women aged 15–44 years). (*From* Guttmacher Institute. Despite recent declines, unintended pregnancy rates in the U.S. remain high among women of color, Infographic. New York: Guttmacher Institute; 2016. Available at: https://www.guttmacher.org/infographic/2016/despite-recent-declines-unintended-pregnancy-rates-us-remain-high-among-women-color; with permission.)

it unintended. Therefore, women trying to prevent "a blessing {they} can't afford" while simultaneously being joyful about it is common.[16]

Aside from pregnancy intention, pregnancy planning is an additional factor in considering what unintended pregnancy is and how women conceive of it. Many women feel that they lack control over pregnancy, reporting it as something that just happens.[11] Both quantitative and qualitative data support the idea that many low-income women see relationship stability and economic security as being necessary for pregnancy planning.[10,11] However, for these women, systems of inequality and disenfranchisement may make these goals difficult to attain, thereby making pregnancy planning out of line with their social circumstances.

For other women, ambivalence or lack of agency around pregnancy may not be caused by structural constraints but may be intentional. Women may think that pregnancy should be a spontaneous process. For some women, pregnancy planning may not seem socially or culturally acceptable. Thus, for many women, the idea of a planned or intended pregnancy may not fit within their perceptions of when and how pregnancy happens.

Given these seeming discrepancies in how unintended pregnancy is defined, how women experience it, and the growing understanding of disparities in health care, perhaps it is time for the approach to pregnancy intendedness and family planning to be reassessed, especially in the clinical encounter. Developing a truly patient-centered approach to family planning, with the patients' wishes and preferences at the forefront, may lead clinicians in the right direction. A patient-centered approach to family planning needs to be broad. It should embrace the concept of family in its fullest sense; – that is, that family may not always be defined as it has been traditionally. It needs to take into consideration that women (and men) may want to plan a pregnancy but think that they will never have the economic stability they want to achieve before doing so. It also needs to take into account that pregnancy ambivalence, even in the context of access to all resources, will still be prevalent and is not necessarily a problem. In addition, it needs to be sensitive to the fact that not everyone wants to plan pregnancy. If able to encompass this breadth, this patient-centered approach, which some describe as reproductive life planning, puts women at the forefront and tries to help them optimize their reproductive choices, whatever they may be.

PRACTICAL, PATIENT-CENTERED APPROACH TO OPTIMIZING REPRODUCTIVE CHOICES
The Complexities of the Patient-Provider Relationship

To establish a patient-centered approach to optimizing reproductive choices, providers need to approach clinical encounters with a patient-centered mindset, understanding the complex dynamics that govern that interaction. The patient-provider clinical encounter is a complex entity that is affected not only by the patient's cultural, ethnic, racial, and social background but by the clinician's as well.[17] In all specialties of medicine, the interplay of these often disparate demographics can affect patients' experiences of the health care encounter, including their ability and willingness to disclose relevant health information. They can also affect the provider's communication behaviors, diagnosis, and treatment.[18–20]

The patient-provider encounter is especially complex in reproductive and sexual health counseling. Cultural norms regarding sexual behavior, childbearing, and motherhood are often not consciously acknowledged by either party, but are inherently part of the encounter. The historical context of coercion within family planning programs can influence both providers and patients.[21] Evidence shows that patient demographics influence the interpersonal interaction with providers in this context. For example, black women report lower satisfaction with clinical encounters and perceive coercion to limit their family size or use a different form of contraception.[22,23] In one survey, two-thirds of black women reported having experienced race-based discrimination when receiving family planning care.[23] In addition, it seems that providers are more likely to agree to sterilize[24,25] and to recommend intrauterine contraception to low-income and nonwhite patients.[26] These findings are concerning, because they suggest that recommendations around fertility goals and contraceptive options, whether permanent or reversible, may be based on patient demographics rather than individual preferences. These findings also imply that nonwhite patients may experience lower quality reproductive health care. This is particularly important because, when patients are given their choice of contraception and receive higher quality of care, they have better contraceptive outcomes.[27,28]

Unlike many other medical conditions in which there is one medically preferred treatment of all patients, the treatment for the prevention of an unintended pregnancy is not circumscribed in this way, nor is the ideal family size. Clinicians discussing reproductive hopes and providing contraception do not have an evidence-based algorithm that dictates what type of birth control should be given to whom. Unlike internists prescribing antihypertensive medications, clinicians tailor their counseling and recommendations to each patient, based on her past experiences and preferences. Therefore, in order not to fall prey to any unconscious bias or unintentional/patient-perceived coercive counseling practices, clinicians should strive to provide truly patient-centered care.

Given the history of reproductive coercion, the potential for unintentional provider bias, and that the perceived quality of the clinical encounter seems to be associated with better outcomes, patient-centered counseling around reproductive preferences is crucial. Although research examining the components of a high-quality visit regarding family planning and contraception is limited, there are some specific steps providers can take to ensure they are providing evidence-based, patient-centered, noncoercive counseling around optimizing reproductive preferences.

Develop a Therapeutic Relationship

Most clinical encounters take place within an already short time frame of approximately 20 minutes.[29] Although time constraints may make it seem more challenging to implement a patient-centered approach, it is possible by incorporating these ideas into a practice.[30]

Establish continuity of care

Although it has not been directly evaluated within the family planning context, within chronic disease management, continuity of care has been found to improve outcomes and patient satisfaction. Although being at risk for unintended pregnancy is not a chronic disease, women may spend three decades of their lives trying to prevent pregnancy. Developing continuity of care allows trust to grow within patient-provider relationships. For some patients, especially those wary of provider-initiated methods of contraception such as implants and intrauterine devices (IUDs), repeated visits with a provider may make such a method more acceptable, because it gives women the reassurances that they will have ongoing care and access to their providers should they desire removal. This increased trust gained through continuity may also allow more honest conversations about pregnancy ambivalence or uncertainty in a way that is respectful of patients' preferences but also allows the transmission of important preconception health information and management of chronic conditions.

Earn patient trust

In order for patients to disclose complete, honest, and highly sensitive information regarding their reproductive health histories and preferences, they assume a vulnerable role in an encounter with an inherent power imbalance, whether because of being a patient, having demographic differences with the physician, or both. Part of assuming this vulnerable role requires trusting that, despite this power imbalance, their physicians will treat them with respect and provide nonjudgmental and comprehensive care and counseling. Demographic differences between patient and provider exacerbate that imbalance, as is well documented by the growing body of literature on health care disparities in the United States.[31,32] Across all fields of medicine, there is clear evidence that patients have better health outcomes when they have high trust in their providers.[33,34] So how do physicians show that they are trustworthy? Unexpectedly, trust is gained not in what physicians say, but by how they say it. Studies show that, when verbal and nonverbal communication from physicians do not match in sincerity, it is the nonverbal communication that patients take as sincere.[35] It is not the words alone, but the actions and nonverbal cues that accompany them. Therefore, basic bedside manners, including a warm handshake and consistent eye contact, can go far in establishing a therapeutic relationship that may improve long-term outcomes.

Acknowledge different values around childbearing

The decision to, or not to, start a family is one of the most personal decisions people make and is driven by personal, cultural, and religious values. Starting a family outside of marriage may be perfectly natural to some but seems irresponsible and misguided to others. Contraceptive decision making is similarly driven by people's personal circumstances. In the United States, among women at risk for unintended pregnancy, use of highly effective, long-acting reversible contraception (LARC) is almost 12%[36] compared with moderately effective methods like the oral contraceptive pill (23%).[37] Contrast this with studies showing that family planning providers use LARC methods, specifically the IUD, at much higher rates, with one convenience sample of family planning fellowship–trained doctors reporting 40% use of IUDs.[38]

Although these highly discrepant IUD use rates may seem like a problem, they most likely reflect differences in values around childbearing and should not be judged or considered in need of correcting. For women to become successful physicians, it is often necessary for them to tightly control their fertility. However, for many professions this is not the case. By acknowledging this difference in values and circumstances driving childbearing decisions, clinicians can avoid the perception by their patients that they are pushing them to use certain types of contraception rather than others and let their values, not ours, guide their choices around fertility and contraception.

Inquire About Reproductive Preferences

Once a therapeutic relationship has been established, how does the clinician explicitly enter a discussion around optimizing reproductive preferences? There are many different options for raising these questions, most of which come under the rubric of reproductive life planning. Current models include the Centers for Disease Control and Preventions Reproductive Life Planning Tool[39] (as well as modified versions of it), One Key Question,[40] and the Reproductive Health Self-assessment Tool (**Table 1**).[41] These tools have not been evaluated side by side in a randomized controlled trial. However, initial studies of acceptability across a wide group of patients suggest that women (and their providers) find value in the process.[41–43] If used in a patient-centered way, these tools leave space for the ambiguity or ambivalence that many women may feel or express around reproductive preferences and child bearing.

Many clinicians encounter patients on a daily basis who decline contraception. Their reasons may be a stated desire to conceive, or an acceptance (either passive or active) that they may conceive without contraception. Each of these women may benefit from fertility or preconception education. Most women are not aware of the benefits of medical planning for a pregnancy[10] and are also unaware of the health value for both themselves and their future pregnancies of obtaining

Table 1
Reproductive life planning tools

Tool	Goal	How It Works	More Information
Reproductive Life Plan Tool for Health Professionals	Screen for reproductive intentions and risks of conceiving	Uses open-ended and branching questions, encourages action steps	http://www.cdc.gov/preconception/rlptool.html
One Key Question	Ensure that pregnancies are wanted, planned, and as healthy as possible	"Would you like to become pregnant in the next year?" Based on response, offer preconception care or contraceptive services	http://www.onekeyquestion.org
RH-SAT	Patient-initiated assessment of reproductive goals	Patients consider their reproductive goals and review additional questions to clarify their intentions	Bello et al,[41] 2013

Abbreviation: RH-SAT, Reproductive Health Self-assessment Tool.

preconception care.[44] Thus, an encounter such as this is an ideal opportunity for effective health education. Discussing the value of preconception care in the context of things women can do to optimize their health can be a positive message for women who are excited to get pregnant or those with striking ambivalence (**Box 1**). Moreover, there is the possibility of benefit for any woman, whether she conceives or not, intentionally or not.

Direct Contraception Counseling

For women who have expressed not only childbearing goals that include delay but also interest in discussing contraception, here are the evidence-based steps that effective contraception counseling should include.

Ask about patient preferences

Contraception use is a preference-driven decision, so the patient's preferences need to be at the forefront. One aspect of contraception use that has recently come to the attention of researchers is the trade-off that women are willing to take in terms of efficacy and side effects. Although there are many forms of birth control, none of them are completely free of side effects. Even the levonorgestrel intrauterine system, a favorite among many providers, has the well-known and sometimes unwelcome side effect of amenorrhea. There are many features of contraceptive methods that women consider to be important. The most commonly described by women at high risk of unintended pregnancy are efficacy, side effects, affordability, ease of use, and being woman-controlled. Women also report that few methods combine all of their preferences, requiring trade-offs.[45] Some data suggest that these preferences may vary by patient race and ethnicity, most likely in part because of a complex history of contraceptive coercion and abuse in communities of color.[46] So how can clinicians elicit their patient's preferences? Here are some options that work:

> *You told me that you stopped using Depo because you didn't get your period. Is having a birth control method in which you get your period important to you? If so, can I discuss with you some methods that would allow for you to get your period and prevent pregnancy?*

> *You mentioned that you got pregnant on pills because you had trouble getting to the drug store every month to pick up a new pack. We could definitely prescribe three packs at a time, but would you also be interested in hearing about methods that don't require you to do much after they are inserted?*

Box 1
Benefits of medical planning of pregnancy

Optimization of chronic conditions

Discontinuation of teratogenic medications

Cessation of unhealthy habits
- Smoking
- Excessive caffeine use

Initiation of healthy habits
- Taking prenatal vitamins
- Practicing good sleep hygiene
- Eating a healthy diet
- Exercising

Talk about the proper use of contraceptive methods
Although there are many benefits to highly effective methods, more than a quarter of women using contraception in the United States end up using a patient-controlled method like the pill, vaginal ring, or contraceptive patch.[37] Given this popularity, it is crucial that providers take the time during contraceptive counseling encounters to review proper use and contingency plans if misuse occurs (including provision of emergency contraception). In addition, providers should maximize their patients' access to these patient-controlled methods. Simply prescribing a several-month supply at a time, as opposed to making a patient go to the drug store monthly, has been associated with higher rates of effective pregnancy prevention.[47] Moreover, in healthy patients for whom patient-controlled methods are low risk, there is no need to hold them hostage to an annual examination for a pill refill. As with initiation,[48] continuation of these methods does not require a pelvic examination.

AREAS FOR FURTHER WORK

Clinicians have numerous tools and techniques at their disposal to help care for underserved women, whose reproductive preferences have frequently been the objects of external control. Recognizing this history and the ongoing health disparities that exist, clinicians are also compelled to look beyond their clinical work and consider research and policy-oriented approaches to address these issues. Some of those possibilities are reviewed here.

Future Research

Reconsidering how clinicians use the term unintended pregnancy
Unintended pregnancy rates continue to be used widely in research as an indicator of women's reproductive health status and access to family planning care. Although this is an important reflection on some aspects of women's reproductive health, it is unclear whether clinicians fully understand what is being measured or whether it is providing a complete picture. From a patient perspective, classification of a pregnancy as unintended is retrospective and may not accurately describe pregnancy intentions. Even without the distorting lens of time, classification of pregnancies is difficult, because many women do not naturally perceive pregnancy intentions in the structure of intended, mistimed, or unwanted.[49] Instead, women perceive pregnancy intention as a response to discovering a pregnancy[13,50] and few spontaneously use words like planned or intended.

Inherent in this metric, or how it has been applied, is the assumption that some pregnancies (those that are unintended) are problems, whereas others (planned pregnancies) are acceptable. Women may not perceive their unintended pregnancies as a problem. Although they may perceive a time when pregnancy would be more ideal, a pregnancy may represent an alternative rather than a problem.[49] Adding to this complicated dynamic is the fact that women of color or women of low socioeconomic status disproportionately experience unintended pregnancies. In addition, the relationship between reported pregnancy intentions and contraceptive behaviors is often discordant. Thus, perhaps clinicians need to reconsider what they are capturing when they measure unintended pregnancy, and what it is they want to measure. An approach that incorporates patients' perceptions of their pregnancies, influenced by their individual needs and social norms, may more accurately represent the complex concept of unintended pregnancy and reproductive preferences.

Further research exploring how patients perceive unintended pregnancy in the context of social norms is needed to develop patient-centered health indicators around reproductive preferences. Use of such indicators may more accurately reflect the true reproductive health of a community. Examples to consider for further research directions include:

- Comparing qualities associated with the planned pregnancy between communities
- Exploring how pregnancy intention and response to discovering a pregnancy changes over the lifespan
- Examining different fertility norms and their roots among communities
- Applying an intendedness framework to other health decisions that may require intention or planning

Exploring Patient-centered Approaches to Optimize Reproductive Preferences

Assessing fertility goals and contraceptive counseling is essential to eliciting patients' reproductive preferences. However, how to best assess fertility goals, perhaps with reproductive life planning tools, is not well established. In contraceptive counseling, even if specific counseling strategies may result in higher uptake of contraception or use of more effective methods, women's choice of contraception is ultimately a preference-driven decision. Contraceptive preference includes understanding how women rank different properties associated with a contraceptive method (side effects, reversibility, use, sexually transmitted infection prevention, cost) to make a decision regarding contraceptive choice. Although most research has focused on method uptake, focusing on preferences may improve overall contraceptive use and continuation.

Fertility goals and contraceptive decision making are different from other medical decisions in that the final decision is largely patient driven. Thus counseling methods must also be driven by patient preference.

Examples to consider for further research directions include:

- Evaluating patient preferences around how to introduce reproductive life planning or other assessments of reproductive goals into clinical encounters
- Examining patient contraception preferences through discrete choice experiments
- Tailoring family planning counseling and tools to be preference based
- Assessing the impact of preference-based counseling using patient satisfaction and traditional reproductive health outcomes

Redefining Measures and Outcomes

Reproductive health metrics should be practical, clinically meaningful and patient centered. Traditional measures like contraceptive continuation rates are important but may not adequately capture the patient experience. Adding metrics that include patient-reported outcomes, like satisfaction, creates a more complete and nuanced perspective.

Policy Implications

Increase access to care

Underserved women need access to the full spectrum of health care services, both within and outside the health care system. If part of the goal of a patient-centered approach to reproductive care is to return to women some of the agency they have lost around their reproduction, this needs to be a universal effort. Conversations around reproductive preferences can happen at health fairs, in youth groups, among friends, and within the health care system. Once within the health care system, policies should ensure that reproductive-age women continue these conversations with health educators, advanced practice providers, and clinicians in various clinical settings. Through improved access to care, health is optimized for when pregnancy does occur, whether it is planned or not.

Recognize and address disparities in health care

If clinicians want to develop a truly patient-centered approach to optimizing reproductive preferences, they must recognize the race-based and class-based disparities that exist within health care. They need to acknowledge that the women most likely to experience an unintended pregnancy, as currently defined, are the same women who are most likely to experience disparities in their care. Thus, it is incumbent on clinicians to develop system-level approaches that can begin to deconstruct the systems that support these inequities. Quality indicators and reimbursement policies need to be structured in such a way as to prioritize and even incentivize the minimization and eventual eradication of these disparities.

Adopt a reproductive justice framework in clinical care, research, and public health policies

Reproductive justice is a positive approach that recognizes the intersectionality of women's reproductive autonomy within the larger context of social justice and is especially mindful of how women's reproductive health is inextricably linked to the health and well-being of their families and communities.[51] This framework recognizes that socially marginalized women have the same variation of desires around fertility, which may include having or not having children, but that decisions around these desires are not made in isolation. Socially marginalized women's entire lives, not just their reproduction, are shaped by the world they have to navigate on a daily basis. A reproductive justice framework can help clinicians, researchers, and public health officials place women and their communities at the center, recognizing the full context of their lives to maximize women's reproductive and overall health.

Support reproductive autonomy

Women's reproductive autonomy should remain at the center of defining pregnancy intention. On a policy level, quality-of-care metrics must never infringe on this. Although metrics using unintended pregnancy and contraceptive uptake provide useful information, they should be paired with patient-centered metrics to create a more complete picture. There is no ideal family size, much like there is no goal for LARC uptake. Quality metrics and policies need to balance public health goals around unintended pregnancy while still respecting women's autonomy.

Providers, researchers, and policy makers can all adopt a patient-centered approach to reproductive preferences in an effort to maximize autonomy and reap population-level benefits.

REFERENCES

1. Finer LB, Zolna MR. Unintended pregnancy in the United States: incidence and disparities, 2006. Contraception 2011;84(5):478–85.
2. Henshaw SK. Unintended pregnancy in the United States. Fam Plann Perspect 1998;30(1):24–9.
3. Gipson JD, Koenig MA, Hindin MJ. The effects of unintended pregnancy on infant, child, and parental health: a review of the literature. Stud Fam Plann 2008; 39(1):18–38.
4. Logan C, Holcombe E, Manlove J, et al. The consequences of unintended childbearing: a white paper. Washington, DC: Child Trends Inc; 2007.

5. D'Angelo D. Preconception and interconception health status of women who recently gave birth to live-born infant–Pregnancy Risk Assessment Monitoring System (PRAMS), United States, 26 reporting areas, 2004. MMWR Surveill Summ 2007;56(10):1–35.

6. Tucker M, Berg C, Callaghan W, et al. The black–white disparity in pregnancy-related mortality from 5 conditions: differences in prevalence and case-fatality rates. Am J Public Health 2007;97:247–51.

7. Rosenberg D, Geller S, Studee L, et al. Disparities in mortality among high risk pregnant women in Illinois: a population based study. Ann Epidemiol 2006;16:26–32.

8. Nagahawatte N, Goldenberg R. Poverty, maternal health, and adverse pregnancy outcomes. Ann N Y Acad Sci 2008;1136:80–5.

9. Finer LB, Zolna MR. Declines in unintended pregnancy in the United States, 2008-2011. N Engl J Med 2016;374(9):843–52.

10. Nelson AL, Shabaik S, Xandre P, et al. Reproductive life planning and preconception care 2015: attitudes of English-speaking family planning patients. J Womens Health (Larchmt) 2016;25(8):832–9.

11. Borrero S, Nikolajski C, Steinberg J, et al. "It just happens": a qualitative study exploring low-income women's perspectives on pregnancy intention and planning. Contraception 2015;91(2):150–6.

12. Biggs M, Karasek D, Foster D. Unprotected intercourse among women wanting to avoid pregnancy: attitudes, behaviors, and beliefs. Womens Health Issues 2012;22(3):311–8.

13. Barrett G, Wellings K. What is a 'planned' pregnancy? Empirical data from a British study. Soc Sci Med 2002;55(4):545–57.

14. Moreau C, Hall K, Trussell J, et al. Effect of prospectively measured pregnancy intentions on the consistency of contraceptive use among young women in Michigan. Hum Reprod 2013;28(3):642–50.

15. Schwarz E, Lohr P, Gold M, et al. Prevalence and correlates of ambivalence towards pregnancy among nonpregnant women. Contraception 2007;75(4):305–10.

16. Aiken A, Dillaway C, Mevs-Korff N. A blessing I can't afford: factors underlying the paradox of happiness about unintended pregnancy. Soc Sci Med 2015;132:149–55.

17. Thom DH, Wong ST, Guzman D, et al. Physician trust in the patient: development and validation of a new measure. Ann Fam Med 2011;9(2):148–54.

18. Burgess DJ, Warren J, Phelan S, et al. Stereotype threat and health disparities: what medical educators and future physicians need to know. J Gen Intern Med 2010;25(Suppl 2):S169–77.

19. Saha S, Sanders DS, Korthuis PT, et al. The role of cultural distance between patient and provider in explaining racial/ethnic disparities in HIV care. Patient Educ Couns 2011;85(3):e278–84.

20. Thornton RL, Powe NR, Roter D, et al. Patient-physician social concordance, medical visit communication and patients' perceptions of health care quality. Patient Educ Couns 2011;85(3):e201–8.

21. Stern AM. Sterilized in the name of public health: race, immigration, and reproductive control in modern California. Am J Public Health 2005;95(7):1128–38.

22. Becker D, Klassen AC, Koenig MA, et al. Women's perspectives on family planning service quality: an exploration of differences by race, ethnicity and language. Perspect Sex Reprod Health 2009;41(3):158–65.

23. Thorburn S, Bogart LM. African American women and family planning services: perceptions of discrimination. Women Health 2005;42(1):23–39.

24. Harrison DD, Cooke CW. An elucidation of factors influencing physicians' willingness to perform elective female sterilization. Obstet Gynecol 1988;72(4):565–70.

25. Borrero S, Schwarz EB, Creinin M, et al. The impact of race and ethnicity on receipt of family planning services in the United States. J Womens Health (Larchmt) 2009;18(1):91–6.

26. Dehlendorf C, Ruskin R, Grumbach K, et al. Recommendations for intrauterine contraception: a randomized trial of the effects of patients' race/ethnicity and socioeconomic status. Am J Obstet Gynecol 2010;203(4):319.e1-8.

27. Pariani S, Heer DM, Van Arsdol MD Jr. Does choice make a difference to contraceptive use? Evidence from east Java. Stud Fam Plann 1991;22(6):384–90.

28. Forrest JD, Frost JJ. The family planning attitudes and experiences of low-income women. Fam Plann Perspect 1996;28(6):246–55, 277.

29. Chen LM, Farwell WR, Jha AK. Primary care visit duration and quality: does good care take longer? Arch Intern Med 2009;169(20):1866–72.

30. Dehlendorf C, Krajewski C, Borrero S. Contraceptive counseling: best practices to ensure quality communication and enable effective contraceptive use. Clin Obstet Gynecol 2014;57(4):659–73.

31. Institute of Medicine Committee on UaE. Racial and ethnic disparities in health care. In: Smedley BD, Stith AY, Nelson AR, editors. Unequal treatment: confronting racial and ethnic disparities in health care. Washington, DC: National Academies Press; 2003.

32. Dehlendorf C, Rodriguez MI, Levy K, et al. Disparities in family planning. Am J Obstet Gynecol 2010;202(3):214–20.

33. Thom DH, Hall MA, Pawlson LG. Measuring patients' trust in physicians when assessing quality of care. Health Aff (Millwood) 2004;23(4):124–32.

34. Hall MA, Zheng B, Dugan E, et al. Measuring patients' trust in their primary care providers. Med Care Res Rev 2002;59(3):293–318.

35. Burgess DJ, Fu SS, van Ryn M. Why do providers contribute to disparities and what can be done about it? J Gen Intern Med 2004;19(11):1154–9.

36. Kavanaugh M, Jerman J, Finer L. Changes in use of long-acting reversible contraceptive methods among U.S. women, 2009–2012. Obstet Gynecol 2015;126(5):917027.

37. Daniels K, Daugherty J, Jones J. Current contraceptive status among women aged 15-44: United States, 2011-2013. NCHS Data Brief 2014;(173):1–8.

38. Stern LF, Simons HR, Kohn JE, et al. Differences in contraceptive use between family planning providers and the U.S. population: results of a nationwide survey. Contraception 2015;91(6):464–9.

39. US Centers for Disease Control and Prevention. Reproductive life plan tool for health professionals. 2016.

40. Bellanca H, Hunter M. ONE KEY QUESTION®: preventive reproductive health is part of high quality primary care. Contraception 2013;88:3–6.

41. Bello JK, Adkins K, Stulberg D, et al. Perceptions of a reproductive health self-assessment tool (RH-SAT) in an urban community health center. Patient Educ Couns 2013;93:655–63.

42. Dunlop AL, Logue KM, Miranda MC, et al. Integrating reproductive planning with primary health care: an exploration among low-income, minority women and men. Sex Reprod Healthc 2010;1(2):37–43.

43. Callegari LS, Borrero S, Reiber GE, et al. Reproductive life planning in primary care: a qualitative study of women veterans' perceptions. Womens Health Issues 2015;25(5):548–54.

44. Steel A, Lucke J, Adams J. The prevalence and nature of the use of preconception services by women with chronic health conditions: an integrative review. BMC Womens Health 2015;15:14.

45. Lessard LN, Karasek D, Ma S, et al. Contraceptive features preferred by women at high risk of unintended pregnancy. Perspect Sex Reprod Health 2012;44(3): 194–200.

46. Jackson AV, Karasek D, Dehlendorf C, et al. Racial and ethnic differences in women's preferences for features of contraceptive methods. Contraception 2016;93(5):406–11.

47. Foster DG, Hulett D, Bradsberry M, et al. Number of oral contraceptive pill packages dispensed and subsequent unintended pregnancies. Obstet Gynecol 2011;117(3):566–72.

48. Henderson J, Sawaya G, Blum M, et al. Pelvic examinations and access to oral hormonal contraception. Obstet Gynecol 2010;116(6):1257–64.

49. Kendall C, Afable-Munsuz A, Speizer I, et al. Understanding pregnancy in a population of inner-city women in New Orleans–results of qualitative research. Soc Sci Med 2005;60(2):297–311.

50. Moos M, Petersen R, Meadows K, et al. Pregnant women's perspectives on intendedness of pregnancy. Womens Health Issues 1997;7(6):385–92.

51. Ross L. Understanding reproductive justice. 2006;2016.

Family Planning American Style Redux

Unintended Pregnancy Improves, Barriers Remain

Lauren Thaxton, MD, MBA, Eve Espey, MD, MPH*

KEYWORDS

- Family planning • America • Sex education • Unintended pregnancy
- Health disparities • Contraception

KEY POINTS

- Barriers to reducing unintended pregnancy include inadequate sex education, confusing media messages about sex, cultural attitudes abut sex and young parenting, conflation of contraception with abortion, inadequate health care access, burdensome cotraceptive dispensing practices, and hospital merger limitations on care.
- Approaches to expanding access to reproductive healthcare include advocacy through traditional and social media channels to increase education about sex and contraception.
- Family planning is an essential component of comprehensive women's healthcare; advocacy to improve access is critical in reducing health inequities.

Because this is America. You're supposed to pretend that you don't notice certain things.

—*Chimamanda Ngozi Adichi, Americanah*

INTRODUCTION

The rate of unintended pregnancy in the United States had been stagnant for several decades, hovering around 50% to 51% of all pregnancies. That rate has finally and definitively decreased. In the most recent cycle of the National Survey of Family Growth (NSFG), a survey reported periodically by the Centers for Disease Control and Prevention (CDC), the rate fell to 45% in 2011, compared with 51% in 2008.[1]

Rates of unintended teenage pregnancies, births, and abortions also have fallen. From 2006 to 2014, teenage birth rates decreased 41% (from 41.1 to 24.2 per 1000

The authors have nothing to disclose.
Department of Obstetrics and Gynecology, MSC10 5580, 1 University of New Mexico, Albuquerque, NM 87131, USA
* Corresponding author.
E-mail address: Eespey@salud.unm.edu

teenagers) (**Fig. 1**).[2] Reductions have occurred across all ethnicities, including African American, Hispanic, and non-Hispanic white teenagers. The largest declines occurred in Hispanic teenagers, followed by African American and non-Hispanic white teenagers. Facilitating these changes are concerted efforts to address the social determinants of teenage pregnancy, including review of community-level reproductive health data by stakeholders, greater access to reproductive health services, and availability of teenager-focused and culturally competent health education materials. Additionally, increases in planned pregnancies are caused by improved access to and use of long-acting reversible contraceptive (LARC) methods, top tier in contraceptive effectiveness.[1]

Although rates of unintended pregnancy, teenage pregnancy, and abortion have dropped dramatically, they remain higher than those for comparable countries in Western European countries. US rates are approximately twice those of France and Sweden.[3] Moreover, despite improvement, disparities persist in unintended and teenage pregnancy among certain racial and ethnic groups. Black and Hispanic teenagers had higher pregnancy rates (93 and 74 per 1000 teenagers) than non-Hispanic white teenagers (35 per 1000 teenagers).[2]

The larger picture goes beyond sexual health to broader social determinants. A recent literature review revealed that socioeconomic factors at the individual and community level, unrelated to sexual health, have a profound effect on teenage pregnancy.[4] Such factors as underemployment, inadequate income and education, and growing up in a disadvantaged neighborhood at the low end of income inequality remind us that solutions to teenage and unintended pregnancy require wide-ranging social change with a focus on equity across the various domains.

This article discusses barriers to reducing unintended pregnancy, focusing on societal obstacles to sexual health. Numerous factors may explain the higher rate in the United States, including inadequate sexual education for adolescents, confusing messages from the media, cultural attitudes about sex and young parenting, conflation of contraception with abortion, burdensome contraceptive dispensing practices, and

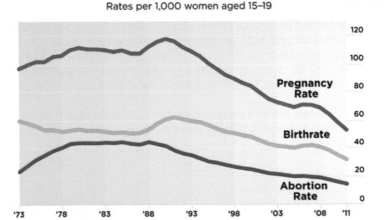

Rates per 1,000 women aged 15–19

Fig. 1. US teenage pregnancy, birth, and abortion rates 1973 to 2011. (*From* Guttmacher Institute. U.S. teen pregnancy, birth and abortion rates reached historic lows in 2011. Infographic. New York: Guttmacher Institute; 2016. Available at: https://www.guttmacher.org/infographic/2016/us-teen-pregnancy-birth-and-abortion-rates-reached-historic-lows-2011; with permission.)

reduced access to health care caused by lack of insurance or hospital mergers. Yet several facilitators can counteract these factors, expanding access to reproductive health care. Local communities and society at large should pursue progressive strategies as a public health priority.

INFLUENCE OF SEXUALITY EDUCATION ON UNINTENDED PREGNANCY

Sexuality education remains a battleground. Beginning in the 1980s and increasing substantially with welfare reform in 1996, significant federal funding promoted abstinence-only-until-marriage education. The federal/state matching program mandated that states receiving federal funding would provide sexuality education that met strict criteria, complying with an eight-item definition of abstinence-only education. The goal of this curriculum is to persuade young people to abstain from sexual activity. It teaches that abstinence is the only certain way to avoid pregnancy and sexually transmitted infections; that sexual activity outside marriage is likely to have harmful psychological and physical effects; and that a mutually faithful, monogamous relationship in the context of marriage is the expected standard of human sexual behavior.[5]

The Obama administration's intent was to end most abstinence-only education programs in favor of comprehensive sexual education, but Congress reinstated $250 million of federal funding for abstinence-only education over a 5-year period. During the last 10 years, taxpayers have supported abstinence-only education programs for adolescents at a cost of more than a billion dollars.[6]

Abstinence-only sex education has been extensively evaluated using such outcome measures as sexual debut, number of sexual partners, effectiveness of virginity pledges, acquisition of sexually transmitted diseases (STDs), and use of contraceptives at first sex. Current research suggests not only that abstinence-only education is ineffective, but also that parents overwhelmingly support comprehensive sex education.[7] Comprehensive sex education that includes abstinence, contraception, and STD prevention seems to optimize reproductive health outcomes.[8-10] Abstinence-only education can do harm: for example, studies of virginity pledges, a common component of several popular abstinence-only education programs, suggest that although pledgers are just as likely to have premarital sex as nonpledgers, they are less likely than nonpledgers to avail themselves of contraception or STD protection.[11] A recent Cochrane review concluded that educational and contraceptive-promoting interventions reduce unintended pregnancy in adolescents.[12]

Evidence strongly supports comprehensive sex education. In 2010 funds became available under the Patient Protection and Affordable Care Act (ACA) for scientifically sound programs that draw on curriculum-based sex education or youth development approaches to prevent teenage pregnancy. Despite mounting evidence of the benefits of comprehensive sex education, the young are less likely today than they were in 1995 or between 2006 and 2010 to receive instruction on contraception.[13] Healthy People 2020 data show a decrease in the percentage of women and men younger than 18 given formal instruction about contraceptive methods. Compared with responses from the 2006 to 2010 period, responses from 2011 to 2013 showed a drop in reported formal birth control education for women from 70% to 60% and for men from 61% to 55%.[13] This reduction is not surprising given the keen focus and massive funding dedicated to abstinence-only sex education over three decades. At coital debut, 79% of female teenagers and 84% of male teenagers used a contraceptive method. Less effective methods, such as condoms, remain the most common contraceptive choice in this age group.[14]

Amid debates on the merits of abstinence-only-until-marriage education versus comprehensive sex education, oddly no federal requirements for the content of sexuality education exist. Some states have created requirements for sex education and human immunodeficiency virus (HIV) prevention but curricula vary widely between states.[15] Whereas 24 states mandate sex education and 18 require information on contraception, 37 states mandate information. Eighteen states require information on contraception and 13 states require that the instruction be medically accurate.

Yet overall despite some state requirements, an analysis of NSFG data showed declines in receipt of formal sex education and disparities between rural and urban areas; adolescents living in nonmetropolitan areas were significantly less apt to obtain instruction in such topics as abstinence, birth control, and STD prevention.[16]

Ironically, despite the inconsistency of sexuality education in the United States, over time some positive changes in teenage sexual activity have occurred.[17,18] From 1995 to 2011 to 2013, fewer teenagers younger than age 15 had become sexually active. From 1982 to 2011 to 2013, more teenagers used contraception at first sex (48% vs 79%). Reductions in formal comprehensive sex education have occurred over the same time period that has seen a drop in teenage birth rates.

Teenagers do not seem to receive additional information from other sources, such as parents or friends; as for social media, its effect is unknown. Although teenage pregnancy rates are lower, widespread adoption of comprehensive sex education has the potential to reduce these rates further. Additionally, a host of professional organizations, including the Society for Adolescent Medicine, the American College of Obstetrics & Gynecology, and the American Pediatrics Association strongly support comprehensive sexuality education, including refusal skills, abstinence, and contraception. The American Academy of Pediatrics (AAP) offered testimony to the House Committee on Oversight and Government reform on behalf of its membership and that of the American Society of Adolescent Medicine, urging funds for comprehensive sex education.[19]

The CDC Healthy People 2020 goals incorporate sexuality education goals, including increasing the percentage of females younger than 18 who receive formal instruction in birth control to 78%, and the percentage of males younger than 18 to 67%. These targets are in alignment with the evidence of the near universality of premarital sex, and of sexual debut by more than half of all women and men by age 18.[17,18] Although age at sexual debut has decreased, common sense dictates that the provision of information for most teenagers who do have sex is bound to have a positive impact on unintended pregnancy and on STD acquisition.

INFLUENCE OF MEDIA ON UNINTENDED PREGNANCY

A disconnect remains between the halting steps toward comprehensive sexuality education and current content of many forms of media, saturated with sex. Although the United States has not embraced comprehensive sexuality education for youth, it has thoroughly adopted the use of sex for advertising a wide range of products. Sexual content also figures large in a range of television shows, from sit-coms to reality television and little of that content conveys messages about responsible sex, including monogamy or safe sex.[20] This schizophrenic approach—to deny in the classroom what is sold in the marketplace—seems distinctly American. We refuse to engage with young people in serious conversations about sex, conversations that could help prevent unwanted pregnancy and STDs and help youth better understand how sexuality may contribute to well-being. Pervasive American morality seems at odds with accepting sexuality as a normal part of human behavior. This leaves many individuals, but particularly youth, confused, with a double standard that creates obstacles to the avoidance of unintended pregnancy.

Americans spend considerable "screen time" between television, mobile devices, and computer use. In 2013 a comprehensive survey studied teenage media use. Two media activities dominated: television and music. The survey found that teenagers use an average of 9 hours of media every day. Those from low-income families use media for considerably more time than teenagers from higher-income families.[21] For "screen" media, lower-income teenagers averaged 8.07 hours a day, whereas higher-income teenagers averaged 5.42 hours.

The potential impact of sexual content on television is important, given the great amount of time Americans spend watching television. In 1998, a total of 56% of television shows contained sexual content, with an average of 3.2 scenes per hour. By 2005, the percentage of shows that included sexual content increased to 70%, with an average of five scenes per hour.[20] Although the Kaiser Family Foundation no longer studies the sexual content of television shows, the Parents Television Council, continues to watchdog content. The Parents Television Council issued a report finding that sexual references in shows had increased by 22%.[22]

Evidence is conflicting regarding the impact of television's sexual content on the sexual behavior of teenagers, although numerous studies attest to the influence on teenagers' attitudes toward sex and on their values and beliefs. A recent study of youth aged 12 to 17 demonstrated a higher likelihood of teenage pregnancy in the 3 years following frequent exposure to television's sexual content including a mix of dramas, comedy, reality, and animated programming.[23] Teenage pregnancy in the high-exposure groups was twice the rate of the low-exposure group, even after adjusting for confounders. Most evidence seems to support an association between more frequent and more sexually explicit viewing as a risk factor for unsafe sexual behavior. These associations led the AAP to publish a strongly worded policy statement directed at pediatricians and the entertainment/broadcast industry.[24] Among the recommendations were these: counseling parents to be aware of and limit teenagers' screen time, encouraging the entertainment industry to produce more programming with responsible sexual content, and urging the broadcast industry to expand airtime for advertising of contraceptives.

Media can also have a positive impact. Several television programs have incorporated positive health-related messaging. Gray's Anatomy and ER dramatized story lines that educated the public about human papilloma virus, emergency contraception, and HIV. In an innovative trial involving social media, messaging was used to increase condom use among at-risk youth. The results showed some evidence of effectiveness.[25] As urged by the AAP, expansion of contraception advertising could have a positive effect on reducing unintended pregnancy. Lack of or highly restricted advertising for contraceptives has been the norm. In the United Kingdom, the AIDS epidemic prompted networks to allow condom advertisements in primetime, rather than confine them to an after 9 PM time slot.[26]

Overall, however, the combination of explicit sexual content in media with limited "responsible" sexuality content or contraceptive advertising constitutes a barrier to reducing unintended pregnancy. Disparities in the consumption of media by lower-income youth may result in additional negative consequences.

CULTURE AND FAMILY PLANNING

Cultural norms may result in unconscious bias that perpetuates negative stereotypes of minority women. In 2011, the birth rate for non-Hispanic white teenagers (21.7 per

1000) was less than half that among non-Hispanic black teenagers and Hispanic teenagers (at 47.2 and 49.6 per 1000, respectively) (**Fig. 2**).[27] This disparity mirrors broader disproportionately adverse health care outcomes occurring within communities of color. Many well-intentioned reproductive health interventions have therefore "targeted" specific communities for an intensive focus on reducing unplanned pregnancy, a practice that can lead to unintended consequences.

Standard expectations for "acceptable" parenting, including age at first birth, family size, and intention to become pregnant, are set by the dominant culture.[28] Members of the dominant culture, high income non-Hispanic whites, are overrepresented in medicine and largely responsible for the reproductive health counseling of young women. Lack of appreciation of the power differential between patient and provider, and cultural biases can unintentionally result in reproductive coercion toward use of contraception and use of specific methods and moral condemnation for reproductive choices and outcomes.[29–31] Although access to contraception may decrease pregnancy, birth, and abortion rates, social determinants may be much more powerful mediators of high birth rates in communities of color. These social determinants involve several inequities experienced daily by members of the nondominant culture.[4] Health care providers must focus on providing knowledge and access to full-spectrum contraceptive options so that women and men are able to make autonomous, well-informed choices grounded in a shared decision-making model.

ACCESS TO CARE: THE IMPACT OF THE AFFORDABLE CARE ACT

Almost every American woman will use a method of contraception at some point in her life (99%). The average American woman spends 30 years preventing pregnancy.[32] Numerous publications appropriately emphasize the cost savings of contraceptive insurance coverage. But even when contraception is "covered," lack of adequate insurance coverage, such as high out-of-pocket costs in the form of copays and deductibles, is a barrier to the affordability of desired methods.

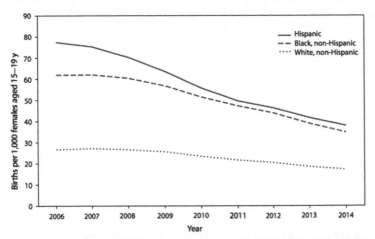

Fig. 2. Birth rates for females aged 15 to 19 years during 2006 to 2014. (*From* Romero L, Pazol K, Warner L, et al. Reduced disparities in birth rates among teens aged 15–19 years— United States, 2006–2007 and 2013–2014. Morb Mortal Wkly Rep 2016;65:411. Available at: http://www.cdc.gov/mmwr/volumes/65/wr/mm6516a1.htm?version=meter+at+null&module=meter-Links&pgtype=article&contentId=&mediaId=&referrer=&priority=true&action=click&contentCollection=meter-links-click. Accessed August 8, 2016.)

The most highly effective reversible methods, intrauterine devices (IUDs) and implants, have high up-front costs despite their long-term cost-effectiveness. In the 2012 NSFG, 11.6% of women reported use of an IUD or implant,[33] a major increase from the prior reporting period, but considerably less than the uptake in many studies of LARC. In the Contraceptive CHOICE study, a large cohort trial conducted in St. Louis, Missouri, 75% of women chose an IUD or implant for contraception when women were offered all methods without financial barriers.[33]

To address the national health care delivery crisis, in 2010 President Obama signed the ACA into law. Based on recommendations from the Institute of Medicine,[34] the Health Resources and Services Administration mandated coverage of "Food and Drug Administration approved contraceptive methods, sterilization procedures, and patient education and counseling for women with reproductive capacity" with at least one form of each type of contraceptive covered without cost sharing.[35]

The impact of the ACA was swift: the proportion of reproductive-aged women who were uninsured fell by 40%. Many women for the first time were able to afford their desired contraceptive method. The number of women who filled prescriptions for birth control pills with no copay exploded, from 1.2 million in 2012 to 5.1 million in 2013.[36] Nationwide claims database research reveals that from 2011 to 2013, the mean copay per contraceptive claim decreased 73%, from $15 to $4. Additionally, the number of commercially insured women with $0 out-of-pocket cost for any contraceptive increased from 10.1% in 2011 to 69.6% in 2013.[37] In 2014, a total of 87% of insured women were able to obtain an IUD without out-of-pocket costs (**Fig. 3** data from the

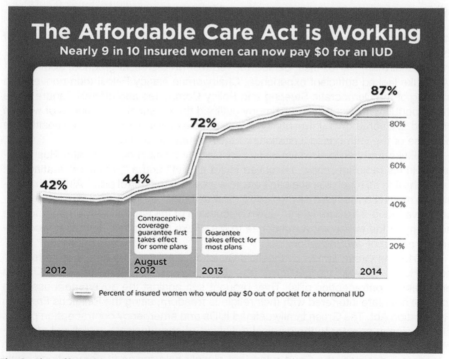

Fig. 3. The Affordable Care Act contraceptive mandate has made contraception more financially attainable for insured women. (*From* Guttmacher Institute. The Affordable Care Act is working. Infographic. New York: Guttmacher Institute; 2016. Available at: https://www.guttmacher.org/infographic/2015/affordable-care-act-working; with permission.)

Guttmacher Institute).[32] By reducing out-of-pocket costs for insured women, the ACA contraceptive mandate has made contraception more financially attainable.

ANTICONTRACEPTIVE POLITICS

Since its inception, the contraception mandate has been mired in religiously motivated activism and anticontraception politics. A vocal minority holds that contraception promotes societal problems, such as promiscuity, an antichild attitude, and the undermining of traditional male-female relationships.[38] Until recently, most experts agreed that improved contraceptive use was a major component in efforts to decrease abortion. A more radical view is that the provider of contraception violates morality. The Catholic doctrine that "every "marital sexual act must be open to the possibility of the transmission of life,"[39] is not supported by the reality that almost all Catholic women have used contraception during their lives.[40] Deplorably, scientific misinformation about the mechanism of action of many contraceptives has led antiabortion activists to oppose several contraceptives. Increasingly, contraception and abortion politics are polarized, partisan topics.[41]

In February 2012, the Republican-led House Oversight and Government Reform Committee organized a hostile review of the ACA contraceptive mandate, claiming it to be an "assault against their freedom of conscience."[42] Specifically, House members asserted that the contraceptive mandate violated the religious freedoms of certain employers whose faith teaches the immorality of contraception. The panel was exclusively composed of male theologians and clergy hearing testimonials from adherents of religious organizations and institutions.

Democratic members of the Committee requested the addition of Georgetown law student, Sandra Fluke, to the list of witnesses. Ms. Fluke had firsthand experience of the difficulties in seeking reproductive health care at a religious university. The Committee Chairman, Darrell Issa, denied the request on technical grounds, adding that Ms. Fluke lacked sufficient experience. Chairwoman Nancy Pelosi then convened a meeting of the Democratic Steering and Policy Committee and offered Sandra Fluke the opportunity to testify. Her testimony outlined the personal experiences of women enrolled at Georgetown University who were unable to obtain full spectrum health care because of the faith-based limitations of their insurance coverage.

Ms. Fluke and her testimonial were criticized by political commentator Rush Limbaugh in his radio talk show. He called Fluke a "slut" and a "prostitute" stating that "she's having so much sex she can't afford her own birth control pills." Although mainstream media condemned his misogyny, "slut shaming" remains a tactic used by conservative thought leaders to shut down discussion of the contraceptive mandate. The acrimony of the conservative response to Ms. Fluke reflects the increasingly controversial nature of contraception.

In 2012, the Green family, Evangelical Christian owners of the arts and crafts business, Hobby Lobby, dropped coverage of two types of contraceptives (IUDs and emergency contraception pills). They brought suit against the government asserting that the mandate interfered with their religious freedom, citing the Religious Freedom Restoration Act. The Green family defined IUDs and emergency contraception pills as abortifacients, counter to the medical definition of abortifacients, which act after implantation. The US Supreme Court accepted the case in *Burwell v. Hobby Lobby*; in a landmark decision, the Court ruled that closely held for-profit corporations could file for a religious exemption to the contraceptive mandate. As Justice Ruth Bader Ginsburg pointed out in her dissent, "the court, I fear, has ventured into a minefield." The implications of this decision are broad insofar as they conflate a critical public health prevention strategy and the interests of women's health with a violation of religious freedom.

HOSPITAL MERGERS

A systems barrier to reducing unintended pregnancy is the negative impact on reproductive health services that occurs when nonsectarian hospitals merge with religious, particularly Catholic, hospitals. In the 10 years from 2001 to 2011, the number of Catholic hospitals increased 16%, more than any other type of nonprofit hospital (**Fig. 4**). Ten of the largest 25 health systems in America are Catholic.[43] In 2016, one in every six acute care hospital beds is in a Catholic owned or Catholic affiliated hospital.[44]

These mergers mean that more and more Americans are being treated in Catholic facilities, which operate under the explicit requirements embodied in the Ethical and Religious Directives (ERDs) for Catholic Health Care Services.[45] Among other services, these directives explicitly oppose abortion, family planning, sterilization of men and women, emergency contraception, and HIV counseling that includes information about condom use. Mergers between nonsectarian and Catholic hospitals often result in the elimination or severe restriction of reproductive health services. In some states, a Catholic owned or affiliated hospital may be the only local hospital.

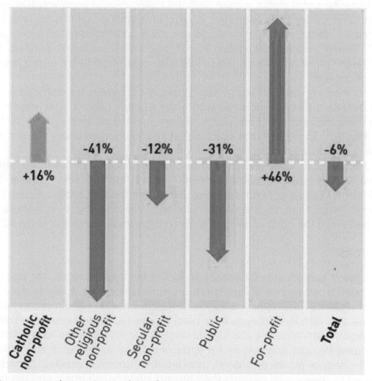

Fig. 4. Percentage change in number of acute-care hospitals by hospital type from 2001 to 2011. (*From* Uttley L, Reynertson S, Kenny L, et al. Miscarriage of medicine: the growth of Catholic hospitals and the threat to reproductive health care. American Civil Liberties Union and the MergerWatch Project. 2013. Available at: https://www.aclu.org/report/miscarriage-medicine. Accessed August 9, 2016; with permission. *Courtesy of* MergerWatch and the ACLU. Artist: Brucie Rosch.)

The impact of the ERD restrictions on reproductive health care should not be ignored. Public activism is a successful strategy. The National Women's Law Center developed the Health Care Provider Merger Project, which uses legal tools to focus attention on the ERD restrictions at the local level.[46] The American Civil Liberties Union recommends national activism to press for investigation into Catholic hospitals for violation of Centers for Medicare and Medicaid Services requirements that all hospitals provide emergency health care regardless of religious affiliation. On an individual level, the American Civil Liberties Union encourages patients to learn whether or not their local hospitals are Catholic run or affiliated and which services are offered.[47]

WHO IS MOST AFFECTED?

Despite the advances in access because of the ACA, certain groups remain at a disadvantage. Objections to ACA coverage of contraception disproportionately affect women already at risk for gaps in coverage including minors, women of color, and women residing in Medicaid nonexpansion states.[48]

Despite professional societies' recommendations to routinely offer highly effective methods, such as IUDs and implants, to adolescents and young women as first-line contraception,[49] uptake remains low. Some postulate that confidentiality may drive nonuse because some states require parental notification of contraceptive services. A 2003 to 2004 survey finds one in five adolescents stating that if faced with mandatory parental notification laws, they would use not contraception at all or rely on withdrawal.[50] Where parental notification is not mandated, teenagers enrolled in their parents' health plans may nevertheless fear loss of confidentiality via explanation of benefits or copays.

Latina women are also less apt to have adequate coverage for reproductive health services despite the ACA. Compared with white women, Latinas have twice the odds of being uninsured and this discrepancy is even more stark among immigrant Latina women (**Fig. 5**).[51] These statistics indicate that institutional and policy barriers are major obstacles to contraception for women of color.

As of July 2016, a total of 19 states have chosen to opt out of Medicaid expansion under the ACA including Alabama, Florida, Georgia, Idaho, Kansas, Maine, Mississippi, Missouri, Nebraska, North Carolina, Oklahoma, South Carolina, South Dakota, Tennessee, Texas, Utah, Virginia, Wisconsin, and Wyoming (**Fig. 6**).[52] In these states, women had twice the odds of being uninsured after implementation of the ACA.

FACILITATORS

Although many barriers impede access to family planning services, the last decade has also seen a resurgence of facilitators promoting women's ability to successfully plan their families. Providers have become more comfortable with an expanded candidate profile and with the techniques for placement of IUDs and implants. The American College of Obstetricians and Gynecologists recommends an expanded profile of candidates thought appropriate for IUDs, including adolescents and nulliparous women.[53] Using a model of shared, nondirective decision making, providers are encouraged to review with patients their reproductive health goals and the range of methods for achieving them.

The American College of Obstetricians and Gynecologists supports other access facilitators, such as same-day initiation of methods, no unnecessary additional medical appointments, and no required pelvic examinations or STD testing before receipt of a method.[54] Medically unnecessary steps create a heavier burden for women seeking

Immigrant women need health coverage, not legal barriers.

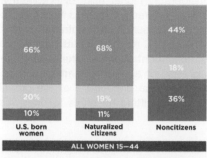

The 6.5 million U.S. women of reproductive
age who are not citizens are much less likely
to be insured...

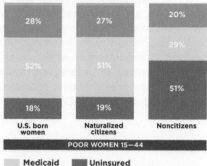

...especially those who live in poverty
and are often barred from Medicaid.

| Other | Privately insured | Medicaid | Uninsured |

Fig. 5. Latina women are less apt to have adequate coverage for reproductive health services despite the ACA. Statistics indicate that institutional and policy barriers are major obstacles to contraception for women of color. *Notes:* Poor women are those in families with incomes under the federal poverty level ($20,090 for a family of three in 2015). Data include some information on undocumented immigrants, although that information is generally acknowledged to be a considerable undercount of that population group. (*From* Guttmacher Institute. Immigrant women need health coverage, not legal barriers. Infographic. New York: Guttmacher Institute; 2016. Available at: https://www.guttmacher.org/infographic/2016/immigrant-women-need-health-coverage-not-legal-barriers; with permission; and Special tabulations of date from the 2016 American Community Survey (data are for 2015).)

Current Status of State Medicaid Expansion Decisions

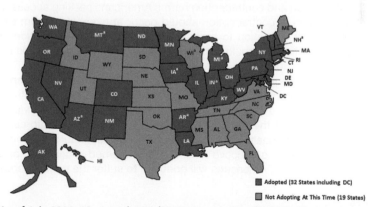

■ Adopted (32 States including DC)

□ Not Adopting At This Time (19 States)

Fig. 6. As of July 2016, 19 states have chosen to opt out of Medicaid expansion under the ACA. *Note:* Current status for each state is based on KCMU tracking and analysis of state executive activity. [a] AR, AZ, IA, IN, MI, MT, and NH have approved Section 1115 waivers. WI covers adults up to 100% FPL in Medicaid, but did not adopt the ACA expansion. FPL, federal poverty level; KCMU; Kaiser Family Foundation's Commission on Medicaid and the Uninsured. (*From* Status of state action on the Medicaid expansion decision. The Henry J. Kaiser Family Foundation. Available at: http://kff.org/health-reform/slide/current-status-of-the-medicaidexpansion-decision/. Accessed August 9, 2016.)

contraception. Another principal facilitator is over-the-counter status for oral contraceptive pills.[55] The greatest risk of oral contraceptives is venous thromboembolism; the argument for over-the-counter status is the rarity of the outcome (3–10.22 per 10,000 women years) compared with the considerably higher risks of pregnancy. Some states, such as California and Oregon as well as Washington and New Mexico now, have passed legislation allowing pharmacists to prescribe oral contraceptives.[56] Immediate postpartum insertion of highly effective LARC methods is also gaining in popularity. The postpartum window is an ideal time for contraception because the patient is known not to be pregnant and she has ease of access to medical professionals.[57,58] In several states, Medicaid has allowed the uncoupling of the global delivery fee from the LARC device and insertion, permitting hospitals to offer this service.

SUMMARY

In 2015, Latin America saw the spread of the mosquito-borne Zika virus. This disease, although typically asymptomatic, is known for the microcephalic babies born to women infected during pregnancy. In the summer of 2016, for the first time, the CDC issued a travel warning to a local city, Miami, Florida, because of a cluster of new cases.[59] The spread of the virus has forced the discussion of reproductive health care in America and of the real-life impact that restrictive family planning and abortion policies create. Although many health experts have indicated that women exposed to the virus should not get pregnant for at least 8 weeks following infection, few policies have translated into actionable plans to meet these reproductive health goals. Systems approaches that focus on education and access to care are critical.[60,61] The ability to prevent the devastating consequences of infection depends on making family planning services available to *all*. Availability is ineffective without education and education alone is insufficient without policy change.

Contraception has become a new political battle ground across the United States and in the nation's capital. American women and families are the victims of this battle; politicization of abortion and contraception harms Americans seeking access to basic health care. Promotion of contraception should occur at every level, from early and comprehensive sexual education to responsible media. Recommendations of religious leaders and politicians should not supersede those made by leagues of health professionals.

Accomplishing health equity starts by recognition that disparities exist. Disparities in reproductive health outcomes based on socioeconomic status and race/ethnicity are compounded by the controversial nature of reproductive health care services. Society's reluctance to accept the reality and impact of reproductive health care needs widens the equity gap. In health care, it is time that Americans turn the spotlight on reproduction. So long as reproductive health care is deemed exceptional or outside of the purview of medicine, Americans will continue to suffer the consequences.

REFERENCES

1. Finer LB, Zolna MR. Declines in unintended pregnancy in the United States, 2008–2011. N Engl J Med 2016;374(9):843–52.

2. Romero L. Reduced disparities in birth rates among teens aged 15–19 years—United States, 2006–2007 and 2013–2014 [Internet]. MMWR Morb Mortal Wkly Rep 2016;65(16):409–14. Available at: http://www.cdc.gov/mmwr/volumes/65/wr/mm6516a1.htm?version=meter+at+null&module=meter-Links&pgtype=article&

contentId=&mediaId=&referrer=&priority=true&action=click&contentCollection= meter-links-click. Accessed August 8, 2016.

3. Advocates for Youth. Adolescent sexual health in Europe and the United States: The case for a rights. Respect. Responsibility® Approach. [Internet]. Available at: http://www.advocatesforyouth.org/storage/advfy/documents/adolescent_sexual_ health_in_europe_and_the_united_states.pdf. Accessed August 1, 2016.

4. Penman-Aguilar A, Carter M, Snead MC, et al. Socioeconomic disadvantage as a social determinant of teen childbearing in the US. Public Health Rep 2013; 128(Suppl 1):5–22.

5. Lerner JE, Hawkins RL. Welfare, liberty, and security for all? U.S. sex education policy and the 1996 title V section 510 of the social security act. Arch Sex Behav 2016;45(5):1027–38.

6. Landor AM, Simons LG. Why virginity pledges succeed or fail: the moderating effect of religious commitment versus religious participation. J Child Fam Stud 2014;23(6):1102–13.

7. Constantine NA. Converging evidence leaves policy behind: sex education in the United States. J Adolesc Health 2008;42(4):324–6.

8. Santelli J, Ott MA, Lyon M, et al. Abstinence and abstinence-only education: a review of U.S. policies and programs. J Adolesc Health 2006;38(1):72–81.

9. Kirby D, Kirby D, National Campaign to Prevent Teen and Unplanned Pregnancy (U.S.). Emerging answers, 2007: research findings on programs to reduce teen pregnancy and sexually transmitted diseases. Washington, DC: National Campaign to Prevent Teen and Unplanned Pregnancy; 2007.

10. Kirby DB, Laris BA, Rolleri LA. Sex and HIV education programs: their impact on sexual behaviors of young people throughout the world. J Adolesc Health 2007; 40(3):206–17.

11. Rosenbaum JE. Patient teenagers? a comparison of the sexual behavior of virginity pledgers and matched nonpledgers. Pediatrics 2009;123(1):e110–20.

12. Oringanje C, Meremikwu MM, Eko H, et al. Interventions for preventing unintended pregnancies among adolescents. In: The Cochrane Collaboration, editor. Cochrane database of systematic reviews. Chichester (United Kingdom): John Wiley & Sons, Ltd; 2016 [Internet]. Available at: http://doi.wiley.com/10.1002/ 14651858.CD005215.pub3. Accessed August 8, 2016.

13. HP2020 Objective Data Search Healthy People 2020. [Internet]. Available at: https://www.healthypeople.gov/2020/data-search/Search-the-Data/page/2/0?nid=& items_per_page=10&pop=&ci=&se=&f%5B%5D=field_topic_area%3A3521. Accessed August 8, 2016.

14. Martinez G, Abma JC. Sexual activity, contraceptive use, and childbearing of teenagers aged 15-19 in the United States [Internet]. NCHS Data Brief 2015;(209):1–8. Available at: http://citeseerx.ist.psu.edu/viewdoc/download? doi=10.1.1.708.4146&rep=rep1&type=pdf. Accessed August 8, 2016.

15. State Policies in Brief: Sex and HIV education. [Internet]. Guttmacher Institute. Available at: https://www.guttmacher.org/view-mode/iframe/26268. Accessed August 1, 2016.

16. Lindberg LD, Maddow-Zimet I, Boonstra H. Changes in adolescents' receipt of sex education, 2006–2013. J Adolesc Health 2016;58(6):621–7.

17. Finer LB, Philbin JM. Sexual initiation, contraceptive use, and pregnancy among young adolescents. Pediatrics 2013;131(5):886–91.

18. Martinez G, Copen C, Abma J. Teenagers in the United States: sexual activity, contraceptive use, and childbearing, 2006–2010 national survey of family growth. Vital Health Stat 23 2011;(31):1–35.

19. Testimony of Margaret J. Blythe MD, FAAP, FSAM on behalf of the American Academy of Pediatrics. [Internet]. Sect. Committee on Oversight and Government Reform Apr 23, 2008. Available at: https://www.aap.org/en-us/advocacy-and-policy/federal-advocacy/Documents/TestimonyofMargaretJ.BlytheMDFAAPFSAM onBehalfoftheAAP.pdf.
20. Collins RL, Elliott MN, Berry SH, et al. Watching sex on television predicts adolescent initiation of sexual behavior. Pediatrics 2004;114(3):e280–9.
21. The Common Sense Census: media use by tweens and teens common sense media. [Internet]. Available at: https://www.commonsensemedia.org/research/the-common-sense-census-media-use-by-tweens-and-teens. Accessed August 8, 2016.
22. Sex on TV is ok as long as it's not safe news - AdAge. [Internet]. Available at: http://adage.com/article/news/sex-tv-long-safe/120489/. Accessed August 8, 2016.
23. Chandra A, Martino SC, Collins RL, et al. Does watching sex on television predict teen pregnancy? Findings from a national longitudinal survey of youth. Pediatrics 2008;122(5):1047–54.
24. American Academy of Pediatrics: committee on psychosocial aspects of child and family health and committee on adolescence. Sexuality education for children and adolescents [Internet]. Pediatrics 2001;108(2):498–502. Available at: http://pediatrics.aappublications.org/content/pediatrics/108/2/498.full.pdf. Accessed August 21, 2016.
25. Bull SS, Levine DK, Black SR, et al. Social media–delivered sexual health intervention. Am J Prev Med 2012;43(5):467–74.
26. Condom TV ads get prime-time all-clear Advertising News the Independent. [Internet]. Available at: http://www.independent.co.uk/news/media/advertising/condom-tv-ads-get-prime-time-all-clear-1922379.html. Accessed August 8, 2016.
27. Kost K, Maddow-Zimet I. U.S. teenage pregnancies, births and abortions, 2011: national trends by age, race and ethnicity. Guttmacher Institute; 2016. Available at: https://www.guttmacher.org/report/us-teen-pregnancy-state-trends-2011.
28. Barber JS, Yarger JE, Gatny HH. Black-white differences in attitudes related to pregnancy among young women. Demography 2015;52(3):751–86.
29. Geronimus AT. Damned if you do: culture, identity, privilege, and teenage childbearing in the United States. Soc Sci Med 2003;57(5):881–93.
30. Borrero S, Nikolajski C, Steinberg JR, et al. "It just happens": a qualitative study exploring low-income women's perspectives on pregnancy intention and planning. Contraception 2015;91(2):150–6.
31. Shreffler KM, Greil AL, Mitchell KS, et al. Variation in pregnancy intendedness across U.S. women's pregnancies. Matern Child Health J 2015;19(5):932–8.
32. Contraception. [Internet]. Guttmacher Institute. Available at: https://www.guttmacher.org/united-states/contraception. Accessed August 8, 2016.
33. Parks C, Peipert JF. Eliminating health disparities in unintended pregnancy with long-acting reversible contraception (LARC). Am J Obstet Gynecol 2016;214(6):681–8.
34. Rosenstock L. Clinical preventive services for women closing the gaps. National Academy of Sciences; 2011. Available at: https://www.nationalacademies.org/hmd/~/media/Files/Report%20Files/2011/Clinical-Preventive-Services-for-Women-Closing-the-Gaps/preventiveservicesforwomenreportbrief_updated2.pdf. Accessed August 8, 2016.
35. Cartwright-Smith L, Rosenbaum S. Controversy, contraception, and conscience: insurance coverage standards under the patient protection and Affordable Care Act. Public Health Rep 2012;127(5):541.

36. IMS Institute for Healthcare Informatics. Medicine use and shifting costs of health-care. [Internet]. 2014. Available at: http://www.plannedparenthoodadvocate.org/2014/IIHI_US_Use_of_Meds_for_2013.pdf. Accessed August 13, 2016.

37. Law A, Wen L, Lin J, et al. Are women benefiting from the affordable care act? A real-world evaluation of the impact of the Affordable Care Act on out-of-pocket costs for contraceptives. Contraception 2016;93(5):392–7.

38. Charo RA. The supreme court decision in the hobby lobby case: conscience, complicity, and contraception. JAMA Intern Med 2014;174(10):1537–8.

39. Zimmer EA, Welie JV, Rendell MS. Copia autorizada por CDR. JAMA 2013; 309(19):1999.

40. Guttmacher statistic on Catholic women's contraceptive use [Internet]. Gutt-macher Institute; 2012. Available at: https://www.guttmacher.org/article/2012/02/guttmacher-statistic-catholic-womens-contraceptive-use. Accessed August 8, 2016.

41. Aiken ARA, Scott JG. Family planning policy in the United States: the converging politics of abortion and contraception. Contraception 2016;93(5):412–20.

42. Lines Crossed: Separation of church and state. Has the Obama Administration trampled on freedom of religion and freedom of conscience? [Internet]. United States House Committee on Oversight and Government Reform. Available at: https://oversight.house.gov/hearing/lines-crossed-separation-of-church-and-state-has-the-obama-administration-trampled-on-freedom-of-religion-and-freedom-of-conscience/. Accessed August 8, 2016.

43. Miscarriage of Medicine. [Internet]. American Civil Liberties Union. Available at: https://www.aclu.org/report/miscarriage-medicine. Accessed August 9, 2016.

44. Uttley L, Khaikin C. Growth of Catholic hospitals and health systems: 2016 update of the Miscarriage of Medicine Report. [Internet]. Available at: http://static1.1.sqspcdn.com/static/f/816571/27061007/1465224862580/MW_Update-2016-MiscarrOfMedicine-report.pdf?token=2OspR0GVZtbKE%2BU1GRn2%2FQInK%2Bs%3D. Accessed August 13, 2016.

45. White KA. Crisis of conscience: reconciling religious health care providers' beliefs and patients' rights. Stanford Law Rev 1999;51(6):1703–49.

46. National Women's Law Center. Health care provider mergers and the threat to women's health services: using certificate of need laws to fight back. [Internet]. Available at: https://nwlc.org/wp-content/uploads/2015/08/Certificate_of_Need_June2002.pdf. Accessed August 13, 2016.

47. Health Care Denied. [Internet]. American Civil Liberties Union. Available at: https://www.aclu.org/feature/health-care-denied. Accessed August 13, 2016.

48. Jones RK, Sonfield A. Health insurance coverage among women of reproductive age before and after implementation of the Affordable Care Act. Contraception 2016;93(5):386–91.

49. Committee opinion no. 539: adolescents and long-acting reversible contracep-tion: implants and intrauterine devices. Obstet Gynecol 2012;120(4):983–8.

50. Jones RK, Purcell A, Singh S, et al. Adolescents' reports of parental knowledge of adolescents' use of sexual health services and their reactions to mandated parental notification for prescription contraception. JAMA 2005;293(3):340–8.

51. Health coverage trends among U.S. women of reproductive age varied consider-ably with ACA implementation. [Internet]. Guttmacher Institute; 2016. Available at: https://www.guttmacher.org/article/2016/02/health-coverage-trends-among-us-women-reproductive-age-varied-considerably-aca. Accessed August 9, 2016.

52. Status of State Action on the Medicaid Expansion Decision. [Internet]. Available at: http://kff.org/health-reform/state-indicator/state-activity-around-expanding-medicaid-under-the-affordable-care-act/. Accessed August 9, 2016.

53. ACOG Practice Bulletin No. 121: Long-acting reversible contraception: implants and intrauterine devices. Obstet Gynecol 2011;118(1):184–96.

54. Committee on Health Care for Underserved Women. Committee Opinion no. 615 Access to Contraception. Obstet Gynecol 2015;125(1):250–5.

55. Committee on Gynecologic Practice, American College of Obstetricians and Gynecologists. Committee Opinion No 544: over-the-counter access to oral contraceptives. Obstet Gynecol 2012;120:1527–31.

56. States start to let pharmacists prescribe birth control pills. [Internet]. Available at: http://pew.org/1PRkaDD. Accessed August 10, 2016.

57. Grimes DA, Lopez LM, Schulz KF, et al. Immediate post-partum insertion of intrauterine devices. Cochrane Database Syst Rev 2010;(5):CD003036.

58. Lopez LM, Bernholc A, Hubacher D, et al. Immediate postpartum insertion of intrauterine device for contraception. In: The Cochrane Collaboration, editor. Cochrane database of systematic reviews. Chichester (United Kingdom): John Wiley & Sons, Ltd; 2015 [Internet]. Available at: http://doi.wiley.com/10.1002/14651858.CD003036.pub3. Accessed August 10, 2016.

59. CDC press releases [Internet]. CDC; 2016. Available at: http://www.cdc.gov/media/releases/2016/p0801-zika-travel-guidance.html. Accessed August 9, 2016.

60. Gostin LO, Hodge JG. Is the United States prepared for a major Zika virus outbreak? [Internet]. JAMA 2016;315(22):2395–6. Available at: http://jama.jamanetwork.com/article.aspx?articleID=2514046. Accessed August 8, 2016.

61. National Women's Law Center. Zika virus, reproductive healthcare, and workplace policies. [Internet]. Available at: https://nwlc.org/wp-content/uploads/2016/06/Zika-Virus-Reproductive-Healthcare-and-Workplace-Policies.pdf. Accessed August 9, 2016.

Leveraging Opportunities for Postpartum Weight Interventions

Alexander Berger, MD, MPH[a], Wanda Kay Nicholson, MD, MPH, MBA[b],*

KEYWORDS

- Postpartum • Weight • Interventions • Cardiovascular disease • Disparities

KEY POINTS

- There are no established clinical guidelines for behavioral counseling for overweight or obese women in the postpartum period.
- Current evidence for the effectiveness of postpartum nutrition and physical activity interventions in African American women is limited, due to small numbers of African American participants and the lack of integration of theory-based behavioral components.
- Parallel to efficacy, additional research is needed in translating efficacious interventions into diverse practice settings.
- Conceptual frameworks, such as reach, efficacy and effectiveness, adoption, implementation, and maintenance (RE-AIM) and the Chronic Care Model, can help to facilitate the integration of weight loss (control) interventions into postpartum care.

Based on current estimates, more than 1.4 million overweight or obese women become pregnant each year in the United States.[1–4] Helping women to prepare for postpartum[5,6] and to achieve a healthy weight after delivery[7] continues to be an important challenge for clinicians within the current US model of care. The postpartum period is generally defined as the 6 to 8 week period after delivery. The interconception period refers to the time between pregnancies, including, but not restricted to, the postpartum period.[8] In many clinical trials and public health reports, the interconception period is referred to as the time frame from delivery to 12 to 18 months after the birth of an infant. Throughout this summary, the term postpartum is broadly used to include the standard 6 to 8 week postpartum period and the interconception period.

Disclosure Statement: The authors have nothing to disclose.
^a Department of Obstetrics & Gynecology, Thomas Jefferson University Hospital, 833 Chestnut Street, Mezz, Philadelphia, PA 19107, USA; ^b Department of Obstetrics & Gynecology, Diabetes and Obesity Core, Center for Women's Health Research, Center for Health Promotion and Disease Prevention, University of North Carolina, Chapel Hill, NC 27599, USA
* Corresponding author. 101 Manning Drive, Campus Box #7570, Chapel Hill, NC 27514.
E-mail address: wknichol@med.unc.edu

Obstet Gynecol Clin N Am 44 (2017) 57–69
http://dx.doi.org/10.1016/j.ogc.2016.11.002
0889-8545/17/© 2016 Elsevier Inc. All rights reserved.

obgyn.theclinics.com

POSTPARTUM AS A CRITICAL PHASE OF A WOMAN'S LIFESPAN

The postpartum period may be a critical period for postpartum weight retention, long-term weight gain, and chronic obesity for young women.[3,4] Physiologic changes of childbirth and sedentary behaviors related to parenting contribute to weight retention and weight gain.[9,10] Compared with weight gain during other life intervals, excess weight retained after childbirth seems to be particularly harmful because postpartum weight accumulates centrally rather than peripherally, increasing the risk of developing the chronic disease.[11,12] Although it is well recognized that the time period after delivery represents a unique opportunity[13] to initiate weight management interventions or to continue interventions that began during pregnancy, there are relatively few opportunities for ongoing patient–clinician communication after delivery. Insurance coverage for postpartum or interconception care, including third-party payers and Medicaid, ends at 6 to 12 weeks after delivery. Most postpartum visits occur within a busy clinical practice and center on contraception, lactation, and resumption of the menstrual cycle. Recent estimates show that only 50% of women, independent of socioeconomic status or insurance, return for the postpartum visit,[14] therefore missing an important opportunity for patient–provider communication about important lifestyle modifications after delivery.

Achieving a healthy weight after delivery in women who were overweight or obese before pregnancy should be possible but will require the use of relevant, evidence-based lifestyle interventions.[15,16] Also, given the 1 brief postpartum visit, interventions will need to be widely disseminated to be deemed successful. This article summarizes the importance of interventions to promote postpartum weight loss among African American women, reviews the findings of a systematic review of current evidence on postpartum interventions and current clinical recommendations for postpartum counseling, briefly discusses potential frameworks for research focused on translating postpartum interventions into clinical and community settings, and summarizes current national initiatives on weight loss (control).

OVERWEIGHT AND OBESITY IN AFRICAN AMERICAN WOMEN

Of the 20 million women currently with obesity in the United States, almost 5 million (15%) are African American.[15] African American women are twice as likely to develop gestational diabetes mellitus compared with their white counterparts. Although prenatal weight gain and postpartum weight retention are key factors in the development of obesity in the female population, there can be distinct racial or ethnic differences in the amount of weight retention and sociodemographic factors that affect postpartum weight retention.[16] Average prenatal weight gain in the United States is 12.6 kg with a range of 1.4 to 37 kg. Average weight gain for African Americans can be 2 to 3 times greater than that of white women. Further, there are differences in the pattern of weight gain among African American and white women.[5] The fat composition of weight gain varies among racial groups and is associated with higher risk for development of type 2 diabetes mellitus and hypertension. Whereas the national average for postpartum weight retention is 3.5 kg, the amount of weight retained can be 3- to 4-fold higher (17 kg) in certain populations, particularly African American and low-income women.[6,7] In a national, population-based study, Keppel and colleagues[15] found that 44% of white women retained 4 lb or more following childbirth compared with 63% of African American women. In the Coronary Artery Risk Development in Young Adults (CARDIA) study,[8] African American women in all parity groups retained twice as much weight as white women and had greater increases in the waist-to-hip ratio. Furthermore, there are racial differences in the factors affecting weight loss following childbirth. Data from the Maternal Infant Health Survey found that unmarried status was associated with weight retention among white mothers, whereas parity was the key factor in African American women. Low socioeconomic status and high prenatal weight gain was associated with an increased risk for weight retention for both black and white mothers. However, there are few studies that have identified barriers to weight loss from the mother's perspective. Despite the prevalence of weight retention following childbirth, particularly among African American and low-income women, few weight loss interventions address barriers to weight loss specific to low-income, African American mothers.

GLOBAL RECOMMENDATIONS FOR POSTPARTUM CARE

Global recommendations for postpartum care for overweight and obese women vary widely. The American Congress of Obstetricians and Gynecologists (ACOG)[17] provides general recommendations for postpartum physical activity but there are no current evidence-based guidelines for dietary or exercise interventions and no recommendations in the United States that specifically target women who were overweight or obese before pregnancy (**Box 1**). The most recent recommendation supports the gradual resumption of prepregnancy exercise activities in those women with uncomplicated pregnancies and provides reassurance that moderate physical activity does not interfere with the quality of milk production or neonatal weight. ACOG does not make specific guidelines for nutritional intake but clinicians are encouraged to provide their patients with information about healthy eating and a list of resources is available through the ACOG Resource Guide—Nutrition and Physical Activity to Address Overweight and Obesity (http://www.acog.org).[18–20] Current recommendations in clinical practice are summarized in **Table 1**.

EVIDENCE FOR POSTPARTUM WEIGHT LOSS INTERVENTIONS

Interventions that integrate exercise and dietary changes have been shown to achieve weight loss in middle- and older-aged adults though evidence for their efficacy in postpartum women is limited. These include PREMIER,[16] Well-Integrated Screening and Evaluation for Women Across the Nation (WISEWOMAN),[21] and the National Diabetes Prevention Program (DPP).[15] The paucity of recommendations for postpartum care in the United States may be due, in part, to the small number of clinical trials that compare the effectiveness and safety of dietary and exercise interventions, small sample size, limitations in study design, and a lack of participants that are generalizable to diverse populations of US women. Reducing postpartum weight retention can decrease the proportion of women who develop pregnancy-related hypertension or gestational diabetes in a subsequent pregnancy. Alternatively, if women have completed childbearing, reducing postpartum weight retention can lower the risk of

---

Box 1
Recommendations for postpartum overweight or obesity care in the United States

- Recommend a moderate level of physical activity for 150 minutes per week.
- Provide information and support for healthy eating.
- Encourage behavioral programs.
- Support breastfeeding.

Table 1
National Institute for Health and Care Excellence and American Congress of Obstetricians and Gynecologists recommendations

	All Postpartum Women	Postpartum Women with BMI ≥30
NICE	6–8 wk postnatal check • Ask those who are overweight, obese, or who have concerns about their weight if they would like any further advice and support now, or later. If they say they would like help later, they should be asked whether they would like to make an appointment within the next 6 mo for advice and support. • Provide clear, tailored, consistent, up-to-date, and timely advice about how to lose weight safely after childbirth. • Ensure women have a realistic expectation of the time it will take to lose weight gained during pregnancy. • Discuss benefits of a healthy diet and regular physical activity, • Advice on healthy eating and physical activity should be tailored to her circumstances. For example, it should take into account the demands of caring for a baby and any other children, how tired she is, and any health problems she may have (eg, pelvic floor muscle weakness or backache). • Advise women, their partners, and family to seek information and advice from a reputable source. • Provide details of appropriate community-based services. • Encourage women to breastfeed. Reassure women that a healthy diet and regular, moderate-intensity physical activity and gradual weight loss will not adversely affect the quantity or quality of breast milk. • Provide advice on recreational exercise from the Royal College of Obstetrics and Gynecology ○ A mild exercise program consisting of walking, pelvic floor exercises, and stretching may begin immediately. ○ After complicated deliveries, or lower segment caesareans, a medical caregiver should be consulted before resuming prepregnancy levels of physical activity, usually after the first check-up at 6–8 wk after giving birth. • Emphasize the importance of participating in physical activities, such as walking, which can be built into daily life.	6–8 wk postnatal check • Explain the increased risks that being obese poses to them and, if they become pregnant again, their unborn child. • Encourage them to lose weight. • Offer a structured weight-loss program or a referral to a dietitian or an appropriately trained health professional. • Provide women who are not yet ready to lose weight with information about where they can get support when they are ready. • Use evidence-based behavior change techniques to motivate and support women to lose weight. • Encourage breastfeeding

(continued on next page)

Table 1 *(continued)*	
All Postpartum Women	**Postpartum Women with BMI ≥30**
ACOG • Rapid return to prepregnancy activities is acceptable after an uncomplicated pregnancy and delivery. • Moderate weight reduction after delivery does not interfere with lactation or neonatal weight. • Postpartum exercise may help to reduce postpartum depression symptoms. • Refer to consultation with a weight specialist before the next pregnancy. • Discuss healthy lifestyle behaviors at each visit.	No recommendations based on BMI

Abbreviations: BMI, body mass index; NICE, National Institute for Health and Care Excellence.

long-term metabolic abnormalities or cardiovascular disease. The PREMIER trial was a National Heart, Lung, and Blood Institute (NHLBI)-funded intervention designed for adults with stage 1 hypertension. The intervention was successful in lowering blood pressure and was found to lower weight. The DPP[15] was a clinical study sponsored by the Centers for Disease Control and Prevention (CDC). Subsequent trials have focused on translating these interventions into various settings[22] Administered through the CDC, the WISEWOMAN program[21] provides low-income, underinsured, or uninsured women, ages 40 to 64 years, with lifestyle intervention and referral services in an effort to prevent cardiovascular disease.

A review of clinical trials comparing diet and exercise interventions for the reduction in postpartum weight retention provides insights into the current gaps in knowledge and care as it relates to obesity in childbearing age women. There are multiple fair-to-good quality randomized controlled trials, based on the United States Preventive Services Task Force quality criteria,[23] that assess the use of evidence-based intervention components proven effective in general populations in postpartum women. Twelve trials[24–34] published between 1998 and 2011 are of fair-to-good quality. Eight trials were conducted in the United States and 1 each in Taiwan,[30] Honduras,[25] Greece,[22] and the United Kingdom.[31] The trials also compared different types of interventions using different modes of delivery. Seven trials compared an in-person diet and exercise intervention to standard postpartum care. Three trials compared the effects of exercise interventions to standard postpartum care: 2 were supervised and 1 was self-directed. One trial compared the effect of individual dietetic counseling and facilitated group sessions with standard postpartum care. The mode of delivery of the interventions varied from mail correspondence to in-person individual and group sessions to telephone follow-up.

The enrollment period for the 12 trials ranged from 1 day to 6 months after delivery. The duration of the interventions was 3 to 9 months. No trials included evidence-based intervention components. Only 3 trials reported the percentage of African American participants.[28,32,35] Ostbye and colleagues[28] reported that African American women comprised 45% and 44% of the intervention and standard care groups, respectively. One trial reported 3.5% of the 40 participants as African American women[29]; another trial reported 1 African American woman among 40 enrollees[32]; 2 studies[31,33] included a small number of nonwhite participants but the specific racial or ethnic groups for participants were not reported.

There were inconsistent results among the 7 trials[28–34] comparing the effect of a postpartum diet and exercise intervention to standard postpartum care on weight (**Table 2**). Five trials[29,31–34] reported greater postpartum weight loss among women in the intervention group compared with those in the usual care group. One study reported no statistically significant differences in weight. In the largest trial by Ostbye and colleagues[28] (N = 450), there were no statistically significant differences in mean weight loss between the intervention and usual care groups. Leermakers and colleagues[33] found a statistically significantly higher percentage weight loss (10% vs 5.8%; *P*<.04) among women in the intervention group compared with those in the control group. Also, there were a higher proportion of women returning to their pre-pregnancy weight (33% vs 11.5%, *P*<.05) in the intervention group versus the standard care group. There were no statistically significant differences in abdominal circumference between women in a diet and exercise intervention and those in usual care. In a small trial, Davenport and colleagues[34] reported statistically significantly lower waist-to-hip ratios in women receiving a diet and exercise intervention compared with usual care.

THEORETIC FRAMEWORKS FOR DEVELOPING AND IMPLEMENTING INTERVENTIONS

Translating evidence-based interventions into postpartum care will require innovative delivery models, collaboration among community and health system leaders, and patient engagement. Two well-known models for clinical and community interventions are the reach, efficacy and effectiveness, adoption, implementation, and maintenance (RE-AIM) framework and the Chronic Care Model. These frameworks have been used extensively in the dissemination of primary care-based interventions. Future research on developing and translating interventions into postpartum care may also use these frameworks to develop outcome metrics and process measures.

Reach, Efficacy and Effectiveness, Adoption, Implementation, and Maintenance Framework

The 4 RE-AIM dimensions allow for a standard set of evaluation parameters that can be used to quantitatively evaluate each project. These 4 dimensions can be used to guide planning, development, and testing of population-based interventions for overweight and obese women. Although well-established within the public health community, the RE-AIM framework has broad applicability to the 1.4 million overweight or obese women who become pregnant each year. The RE-AIM framework is particularly relevant to the topic of postpartum weight retention and prevention of obesity because it provides flexibility for clinicians and researchers to modify the framework to relate to their specific target population, recruitment and outreach approaches, efficacy, adoption, implementation, and maintenance. Given the multiple settings in which women may receive care after delivery (private medical office, health department, hospital-based clinic), a general framework that can be modified for specific populations and settings can be useful in designing dissemination studies.

Chronic Care Model

A potential theoretic approach to creating effective postpartum care in the overweight or obese parturient is the Chronic Care Model.[36,37] Building from this model, clinicians and public health officials can rigorously engage other community-based providers, including behavioral interventionists, dieticians, exercise physiologists, and lifestyle coaches to assist patients with the important lifestyle modifications necessary to reach their weight loss goals. The Chronic Care Model is particularly relevant to

Table 2
Results from 12 randomized controlled trials of diet and exercise interventions

Author, Year, Country	Intervention Arms	Intervention Enrollment or Duration	Study Sample, Number (N)	Race or Ethnicity	Weight Change, (kg, Standard Deviation (SD)
Diet Plus Exercise Interventions					
Leermakers, 1998, US[33]	I: Correspondence lessons, group sessions, and telephone follow-up C: Usual care, brochure	8 mo; 6 mo	Nonlactating postpartum women; N = 90	3% Nonwhite	I: −7.8 ± 4.5 C: −4.9 ± 5.4 (P = .03)
O'Toole, 2003, US[32]	I: Structured diet + exercise with weekly in-person sessions × 12 wk, biweekly sessions × 8 wk, and monthly sessions up to 1 y C: 1 session, self-directed	6 wk-6 mo; 6–10 mo	Postpartum women who were overweight or obese before pregnancy; N = 40	1 AA	I: −4.8 ± 1.7 C: −0.8 ± 2.3 (P<.001)
Craigie, 2011, UK[31]	I: 2 face-to-face counseling sessions, with telephone follow-up for reinforcement and resources pamphlet C: Information pamphlet	6–18 mo; 3 mo	Low-income, overweight, and obese postpartum women; N = 52	3 Nonwhite participants	I: −7.3 C: −1.3 (P<.05) SD, NR
Huang, 2011, Taiwan[30]	I: Individualized dietary and physical activity plans, including 6 in-person pregnancy sessions and 3 postpartum sessions C: Usual care	1 d; 6 mo	Pregnant and postpartum Taiwanese women; 1 d postpartum; N = 189	Taiwanese	I: −0.9 ± 5.1 C: −0.36 ± 4.9 (P = .25)

(continued on next page)

Table 2
(continued)

Author, Year, Country	Intervention Arms	Intervention Enrollment or Duration	Study Sample, Number (N)	Race or Ethnicity	Weight Change, (kg, Standard Deviation (SD)
Lovelady, 2000, US[29]	I: Caloric restriction and exercise intervention, including 4 exercise sessions, lasting 43 min with goal of 65%–80% heart rate C: Usual care	5 wk; 2.5 mo	Overweight postpartum women with BMI 25–30 kg/m2, exclusively breastfeeding: N = 40	3.5% AA	I: −1.6 ± 2.0 C: 0.2 ± 2.2 (P = .018)
Ostbye, 2009, US[28]	I: 8 healthy eating classes, 10 physical activity classes, and 6 telephone counseling sessions over 9 mo C: Usual care	2 mo; 9 mo	Overweight or obese postpartum women; N = 450	I: 45% AA C: 45% AA	I: −11.21 C: −11.04 (P-value NR) SD, NR
Davenport, 2011, US[34]	I: Diet + low-intensity exercise I: Diet + moderate-intensity exercise C: No intervention	8 wk; 4 mo	Overweight or obese women who retained >5 kg after delivery; N = 60	Intervention groups: 85%–90% white No AA Other race: NR	I: −5.0 ± 2.9 moderate-intensity I: −4.2 ± 4.0 low-intensity C: −0.1 ± 3.3 (P<.01)
Exercise-Only Interventions					
Zourladani, 2011, Greece[22]	I: Instructor-led 1-h exercise class with aerobic activity and strength training 3 times per wk for 12 wk. C: No intervention	4–6 wk; 3 mo	Primiparous postpartum women; N = 40	Greek	I: −3.3 C: −1.3; (P = 0.667)

Maturi, 2011, Iran[27]	Tailored pedometer-based walking program with baseline counseling session, cellular phone, and text reminders, and telephone feedback; C: Routine care	6wk–6 mo; 3 mo	Lactating, normal or overweight postpartum women; N = 66	Iranian	I: −2.1 C: 0 ($P<.001$)
Dewey, 1994, US[26]	I: Individually tailored and supervised aerobic activity to achieve 60%–70% heart rate reserve; 45 min 5 ×wk C: No intervention	6–8 wk; 3 mo	Exclusively breastfeeding postpartum women; N = 33	No AA	I: −1.6 C: −1.6 ($P>.05$)
Diet-Only Intervention					
Krummel, 2010, US[24]	Counseling with dietitian, 10 facilitated discussion groups, monthly personalized feedback on self-monitoring records C: Self-directed	30 wk; 12 mo	Postpartum women enrolled in WIC; N = 151	10% Nonwhite;	I: −2.1 C: 0 ($P<.001$) SD, NR
Breastfeeding Intervention					
Dewey, 2001, Honduras[25]	I: Received counseling on exclusive breastfeeding C: Usual care	4 mo; 2 mo	2 studies: Postpartum, primiparous, low-income women; N = 141	NR	Cohort 1: I: −0.7 ± 1.5 C: −0.1 ± 1.7 ($P<.05$)

Abbreviations: AA, African American; BMI, body mass index; C, control; I, intervention; NR, not reported; WIC, Women, Infants, and Children program.

reducing postpartum weight retention because it includes condition-specific decision support and general skill building around prevention. Interventions that share success similar to other interventions based on this model have the potential to provide significant improvements in overall health in preparation for a future pregnancy and for long-term health.

FUTURE RESEARCH

Further research is needed to determine the effectiveness of postpartum intervention on weight and measures of adiposity (eg, waist circumference, skinfold thickness) and increase understanding of which single component or combination of components is most effective in postpartum women. Large-scale studies that include a diverse sample of participants, improved adherence to intervention protocol, and consistency in outcome measures can provide better insight into the effectiveness of intervention. Further, studies should include an examination of harms, including effects on both the mother and infant child. Such studies can inform the development of postpartum care guidelines tailored to overweight or obese women. The LifeMoms Consortium,[38] sponsored by the National Institutes of Health (NIH), consists of 6 ongoing large studies of pregnancy and postpartum interventions. The overall goal of the Consortium is to determine effective behavioral and lifestyle interventions that will maximize weight, glycemic control, and other-pregnancy-related outcomes in overweight and obese pregnant women. Findings from these ongoing studies should address some of the existing gaps in current knowledge and inform postpartum care guidelines. As these guidelines are formed, evidence-based interventions will be more easily disseminated to the providers at the front lines of the obesity epidemic.

POLICY IMPLICATIONS

Multiple national, regional, and state initiatives to promote lifestyle modifications among women and their families have grown over the past decade. These initiatives, spearheaded by the White House, CDC, health care organizations, and state health agencies, focus on educating adults about the adverse health consequences of obesity and the importance of healthy eating and physical activity. The long-term goal of these policy initiatives is to increase the availability of low-cost healthy foods, promote safe neighborhood venues for physical activity, and promote knowledge about the caloric and fat content of foods.

INITIATIVES TO PREVENT OBESITY
National Initiatives

The Let's Move campaign,[9] launched by First Lady Michelle Obama, combats child obesity by promoting family-centered interventions. The campaign identifies strategies to create a healthy start for children, empower parents and caregivers in setting an example of healthy eating, advocate for healthy foods in school cafeterias, increase the availability of healthy foods, and promote physical activity. Several subprograms within the Let's Move campaign target adults through faith-based organizations and promote physical activity and regular exercise in particularly high-risk populations, including American Indians and Alaskan natives. The campaign (Let's Move! In the Clinic) promotes professional partnerships between the program and health care professionals.

The DPP,[10] supported by the CDC, is designed to bring to communities evidence-based lifestyle change programs for weight loss and prevention of type 2 diabetes.

The program is based on the DPP research study led by the NIH and supported by CDC. The lifestyle program in this study showed that making modest behavior changes (increasing healthy food choices and physical activity to at least 150 minutes per week), helped male and female participants to lose 5% to 7% of their body weight and reduced the risk of developing type 2 diabetes mellitus. Participants work with a lifestyle coach in a group setting to receive a 1-year lifestyle change program. Current efforts are on translating the program into diverse clinical settings.

REFERENCES

1. Setse R, Grogan R, Cooper LA, et al. Weight loss programs for urban-based, postpartum African-American women: perceived barriers and preferred components. Matern Child Health J 2008;12(1):119–27.
2. Flegal KM, Carroll MD, Kit BK, et al. Prevalence of obesity and trends in the distribution of body mass index among US adults, 1999-2010. JAMA 2012;307(5): 491–7.
3. Gunderson EP, Abrams B, Selvin S. The relative importance of gestational gain and maternal characteristics associated with the risk of becoming overweight after pregnancy. Int J Obes Relat Metab Disord 2000;24(12):1660–8.
4. Gore SA, Brown DM, West DS. The role of postpartum weight retention in obesity among women: a review of the evidence. Ann Behav Med 2003;26(2):149–59.
5. Howell EA. Lack of patient preparation for the postpartum period and patients' satisfaction with their obstetric clinicians. Obstet Gynecol 2010;115(2 Pt 1): 284–9.
6. Martin A, Horowitz C, Balbierz A, et al. Views of women and clinicians on postpartum preparation and recovery. Matern Child Health J 2014;18(3):707–13.
7. Ostbye T, Krause KM, Brouwer RJ, et al. Active Mothers Postpartum (AMP): rationale, design, and baseline characteristics. J Womens Health (Larchmt) 2008; 17(10):1567–75.
8. Available at: www.cdc.gov/nchs/data. Accessed December 5, 2016.
9. Rooney BL, Schauberger CW, Mathiason MA. Impact of perinatal weight change on long-term obesity and obesity-related illnesses. Obstet Gynecol 2005;106(6): 1349–56.
10. Kral JG. Preventing and treating obesity in girls and young women to curb the epidemic. Obes Res 2004;12(10):1539–46.
11. Gunderson EP, Murtaugh MA, Lewis CE, et al. Excess gains in weight and waist circumference associated with childbearing: the Coronary Artery Risk Development in Young Adults Study (CARDIA). Int J Obes Relat Metab Disord 2004; 28(4):525–35.
12. Smith DE, Lewis CE, Caveny JL, et al. Longitudinal changes in adiposity associated with pregnancy. The CARDIA Study. Coronary Artery Risk Development in Young Adults Study. JAMA 1994;271(22):1747–51.
13. McBride CM, Emmons KM, Lipkus IM. Understanding the potential of teachable moments: the case of smoking cessation. Health Educ Res 2003;18(2):156–70.
14. Weir S, Posner HE, Zhang J, et al. Predictors of prenatal and postpartum care adequacy in a Medicaid managed care population. Womens Health Issues 2011; 21(4):277–85.
15. Keppel KG, Taffel SM. Pregnancy-related weight gain and retention: implications of the 1990 Institute of Medicine guidelines. Am J Public Health 1993;83(8): 1100–3.

16. Appel LJ, Champagne CM, Harsha DW, et al. Effect of comprehensive lifestyle modification on blood pressure control: main results of the PREMIER clinical trial. JAMA 2003;289(16):2083–93.

17. ACOG Committee Opinion No. 650: Physical activity and exercise during pregnancy and the postpartum period. Obstet Gynecol 2015;126(6):e135–42.

18. Available at: http://www.acog.org. ARG-NaPAtAOaO. Accessed December 6, 2016.

19. Davies GA, Wolfe LA, Mottola MF, et al. Joint SOGC/CSEP clinical practice guideline: exercise in pregnancy and the postpartum period. Can J Appl Physiol 2003; 28:330–41.

20. National Institute for Health and Clinical Excellence (NICE). Weight management before, during and after pregnancy. In NICE Public Health Guidance 27. London; 2010.

21. Nelson TL, Hunt KJ, Rosamond WD, et al. Obesity and associated coronary heart disease risk factors in a population of low-income African-American and white women: the North Carolina WISEWOMAN project. Prev Med 2002;35(1):1–6.

22. Zourladani A, Tsaloglidou A, Tzetzis G, et al. The effect of a low impact exercise training programme on the well-being of Greek postpartum women: a randomised controlled trial. Int J Sports Med 2011;12(1):30–8.

23. Atkins D, Best D, Briss PA, et al. Grading quality of evidence and strength of recommendations. BMJ 2004;328(7454):1490.

24. Krummel D, Semmens E, MacBride AM, et al. Lessons learned from the mothers' overweight management study in 4 West Virginia WIC offices. J Nutr Educ Behav 2010;42(3S):S52–8.

25. Dewey KG, Cohen RJ, Brown KH, et al. Effects of exclusive breastfeeding for four versus six months on maternal nutritional status and infant motor development: results of two randomized trials in Honduras. J Nutr 2001;131(2):262–7.

26. Dewey KG, Lovelady CA, Nommsen-Rivers LA, McCory MA, et al. A randomized study of the effects of aerobic exercise by lactating women on breast-milk volume and composition. N Engl J Med 1994;330:449–53.

27. Maturi SM, Afshary P, Abedi P. Effect of physical activity intervention based on a pedometer on physical activity level and anthropometric measures after childbirth: a randomized controlled trial. BMC Pregnancy Childbirth 2011;11(10):103.

28. Ostbye T, Krause KM, Lovelady CA, et al. Active Mothers Postpartum: a randomized controlled weight-loss intervention trial. Am J Prev Med 2009;37(3):173–80.

29. Lovelady CA, Garner KE, Moreno KL, et al. The effect of weight loss in overweight, lactating women on the growth of their infants. N Engl J Med 2000; 342(7):449–53.

30. Huang TT, Yeh CY, Tsai YC. A diet and physical activity intervention for preventing weight retention among Taiwanese childbearing women: a randomized controlled trial. Midwifery 2011;27(2):257–64.

31. Craigie AM, Macleod M, Barton KL, et al. Supporting postpartum weight loss in women living in deprived communities: design implications for a randomized control trial. Eur J Clin Nutr 2011;65:952–8.

32. O'Toole ML, Sawicki MA, Artal R. Structured diet and physical activity prevent postpartum weight retention. J Womens Health (Larchmt) 2003;12(10):991–8.

33. Leermakers EA, Anglin K, Wing RR. Reducing postpartum weight retention through a correspondence intervention. Int J Obes Relat Metab Disord 1998; 22(11):1103–9.

34. Davenport MH, Giroux IG, Sopper MM, et al. Postpartum exercise regardless of intensity improves chronic disease risk factors. Med Sci Sports Exerc 2011;43(6): 951–8.
35. Lovelady CA, Nommsen-Rivers LA, McCrory MA, et al. Effects of exercise on plasma lipids and metabolism of lactating women. Med Sci Sports Exerc 1995; 27(1):22–8.
36. Stuckey HL, Dellasega C, Graber NJ, et al. Diabetes nurse case management and motivational interviewing for change (DYNAMIC): study design and baseline characteristics in the Chronic Care Model for type 2 diabetes. Contemp Clin Trials 2009;30(4):366–74.
37. Barr VJ, Robinson S, Marin-Link B, et al. The expanded Chronic Care Model: an integration of concepts and strategies from population health promotion and the Chronic Care Model. Hosp Q 2003;7(1):73–82.
38. Available at: https://portal.bsc.gwu.edu/web/lifemoms. Accessed December 9, 2016.

Addressing Health Care Disparities Among Sexual Minorities

Kesha Baptiste-Roberts, PhD, MPH[a],*, Ebele Oranuba, MBBS, MPH[a],
Niya Werts, PhD, MIS[b], Lorece V. Edwards, DrPH[c]

KEYWORDS

- Sexual minority • Health disparity • Intervention

KEY POINTS

- Sexual minority women, lesbians, bisexual women, and women who have sex with women experience health disparities, and few interventions have focused on this underserved group of women.
- There is limited research on the health status and health needs of the lesbian, gay, bisexual, and transgender population and this research has primarily focused on sexually transmitted infection among men who have sex with men, with little focus on sexual minority women (lesbians, bisexual women, and women who have sex with women).
- Compared with their heterosexual counterparts, sexual minority women are more likely to report poorer mental and physical health and less access to and use of health care services.
- There is a need for cultural sensitivity training for health care providers and health care facility staff to reduce homophobia and heterosexism, which may be harmful/noninclusive of sexual minority women.

INTRODUCTION

In the past decade, there has been significant emphasis on reducing disparities in health, resulting in substantial attention on racial/ethnic, socioeconomic, and gender disparities, but little on sexual orientation disparities. The lesbian, gay, bisexual, and transgender (LGBT) community is becoming more visible in society and there has been substantial progress in the social acknowledgment of the LGBT community. Common terms used in LGBT health are shown in **Box 1**. A recent report by the United

Disclosure: The authors have nothing to disclose.
[a] Department of Public Health Analysis, School of Community Health & Policy, Morgan State University, 4530 Portage Avenue Campus, Suite 211, 1700 East Cold Spring Lane, Baltimore, MD 21251, USA; [b] Department of Health Science, Towson University, 8000 York Road, Baltimore, MD 21252, USA; [c] Department of Behavioral Health Science, School of Community Health & Policy, Morgan State University, 1700 East Cold Spring Lane, Baltimore, MD 21251, USA
* Corresponding author.
E-mail address: kesha.baptisteroberts@morgan.edu

Obstet Gynecol Clin N Am 44 (2017) 71–80
http://dx.doi.org/10.1016/j.ogc.2016.11.003
0889-8545/17/© 2016 Elsevier Inc. All rights reserved.

obgyn.theclinics.com

Box 1	
Common terms used in lesbian, gay, bisexual, and transgender health	
Term	**Definition**
Sexual minority	Lesbian, gay, bisexual, transgender, questioning, queer
Sexual orientation	An individual's pattern of emotional attractions to others (same sex, different sex, or multiple)
Lesbian	Woman who identifies her primary sexual and loving attachments as being predominantly female
Bisexual	Women or men who identify their primary sexual and loving attachments as being with both sexes
Queer	Originally derogatory, now reclaimed to describe individuals who reject mainstream cultural norms of sexuality and gender
Women who have sex with women	A woman who has sexual contact with other women whether or not she identifies as lesbian or has sexual contact with men

States Center for Health Statistics using 2013 National Health Interview Survey (NHIS) data stated that 1.6% of US adults 18 years of age and older self-identify as gay or lesbian and 0.7% self-identify as bisexual.[1] This finding was similar among men and women, except that a slightly higher proportion of women self-identified as bisexual (0.9% vs 0.7%) compared with men. However, little is known about the health status and health care needs of members of the LGBT community. Moreover, most of the research on LGBT health has focused on human immunodeficiency virus (HIV)/acquired immunodeficiency syndrome (AIDS) and other sexually transmitted infections (STIs) among sexual minority men; that is, men who have sex with men.[2] Research on the health of sexual minority women (lesbians, bisexual women, and women who have sex with women) and transgender populations is limited.

In 1999, the Institute of Medicine (IOM) issued a report on lesbian health indicating the importance of identifying and understanding factors unique to lesbians and their impacts on health.[3] Following this report a goal was added to the Healthy People 2020 initiative to improve the health, safety, and well-being of LGBT persons. Later in 2011, the IOM acknowledged that members of the LGBT community have unique health experiences and needs.[2] This report also revealed disparities in several health indicators, such as perceived health status, obesity, smoking, alcohol abuse, and health care access.

This article focuses on health disparities among sexual minority women (ie, lesbians, bisexual women, women who have sex with women [WSW]) and examines community initiatives to address these disparities. Several studies,[4] including combined data from the 2013 and 2014 NHIS, show that lesbian women were more likely to report moderate psychological distress, poor or fair health, multiple chronic conditions, heavy drinking, and heavy smoking compared with heterosexual women. Similarly, bisexual women were more likely to report multiple chronic conditions, severe psychological distress, heavy drinking, and moderate smoking.[5]

These disparities in health among sexual minority women may be influenced by the stressful social environment caused by societal stigma, prejudice, and discrimination, which have been described in terms of minority stress or chronic stress associated with being a member of a marginalized minority group.[6] The minority stress theory has been used frequently to study mental health issues among sexual minority groups[7] and is defined as the excess stress to which individuals from stigmatized social categories are exposed, because of their minority position in society.[8] Although the minority stress model is focused on mental health, there is some evidence to support the extension of the minority stress model to physical health. Meyer[8] describes minority stress processes along a continuum from distal to proximal. Distal stressors are defined as objective events and conditions, whereas proximal events are subjective personal processes because these rely on individual perception. Sources of minority stress may include discrimination, victimization, and negative feelings regarding a person's own sexual orientation; commonly referred to as internalized homophobia. Studies have shown that these sources of stress are associated with poorer mental health outcomes.[9–11] Minority groups often respond to minority stress with coping and resilience. However, mechanisms and sources of coping and resilience may have serious implications for overall health and well-being.

Data for measuring and monitoring the health of LGBT populations in the United States have been limited. Most of the research has been conducted using nonrandom convenience samples from clinic settings or community organizations. Because of small sample sizes, data have been pooled over several years and all LGBT adults have been included in a single category, resulting in challenges for making generalizations or appreciating the diversity within the LGBT community and the unique needs of subpopulations within the LGBT community.

MENTAL HEALTH

There is overwhelming evidence that members of the LGBT community experience poorer mental health than their heterosexual counterparts. Studies consistently show increased rates of mental disorders, substance use, violence, self-harm, and suicidality.[12–14] Using the minority stress theory, these increased rates in poor mental health may be a result of chronic adverse distal and proximal stressors. Similar to what is observed in the heterosexual population, mental health disorders such as depression and mood/anxiety disorders tend to co-occur with heavy drinking and substance abuse. An understudied aspect of minority stress prevalent among sexual minority women is sexual identity mobility. Sexual identity mobility is defined as changes in self-reported sexual orientation and is a major contributor to depressive symptoms.[15] These changes in sexual identity seem to be more common among women compared with men.[16–18] In addition, women are more likely to report changes in their sexual identity later in life.[19]

Postpartum Depression

Research on postpartum depression (PPD) among sexual minority women is limited because most studies do not report on participant sexual orientation. Data from the National Survey of Family Growth indicate that 34.9% of lesbian women and 44.8% of bisexual women have given birth.[20] Between 13% and 19.2% of women experience PPD.[21] Given the minority stress and the confluence of factors during pregnancy, it is possible that a large number of sexual minority women may experience PPD, and several studies report that sexual minority women may be at higher risk for PPD.[22–24] Moreover, Ross and colleagues[22] found that known risk factors among heterosexual women, such as lack of social support and relationship satisfaction, did not explain the increased risk in sexual minority women. Researchers have suggested other factors, like social exclusion, minority stress, and internalized homophobia, as possible contributors to the excess risk. The few studies that have addressed this topic have not explored different subgroups of sexual minority women (lesbians, bisexuals, WSW), although there is some evidence that there are significant differences in mental health outcomes between bisexual and lesbian women, with bisexual women reporting poorer mental health.[25] Given that a history of poor mental health is predictive of PPD, it is important to refrain from assuming homogeneity within the sexual minority group. In one study, women who had sex with individuals of more than 1 gender in the past 5 years, but who were currently partnered with men (referred to as invisible sexual minority women), had higher Edinburgh Postnatal Depression Scale scores compared with women consistently partnered with men. This effect was not found in women who were currently partnered with women or who were unpartnered.[20] These results support the added mental health burden caused by sexual identity mobility among women.

SEXUAL HEALTH

Sexual minority women, especially lesbians, frequently underestimate their risk of acquiring or being capable of transmitting sexual disease, because they consider this most likely to occur in sexual relationships with male partners or heterosexual relationships.[26] In large part because of the AIDS epidemic, much of the lens of sexual health in the LGBT community has traditionally been focused on STIs.[27] However, lesbian women have historically faced barriers to STI testing and treatment because of the perception that they are inherently a low-risk group.[28–30] This perception has been explicitly furthered by some medical professionals[28,29,31] and self-perpetuated within the lesbian community.[30,32] In addition, lesbian and bisexual women have also reported a cognitive distance from safer sex health promotion messages that are often perceived to apply primarily to women who have sex with men rather than women universally.[30] The perception that lesbians or WSW are a low-risk group for STIs is inherently problematic because woman-to-woman transmission of several sexually transmitted infections, including HIV, human papilloma virus, herpes, *Treponema pallidum* (syphilis), *Chlamydia*, *Trichomonas vaginalis*, bacterial vaginosis, and *Candida*, have been documented.[28,29,31,33–35]

Sexual transmitted infection risk for lesbian women and other categories of WSW is also complicated by the failure of sexual orientation identification to consistently align with sexual behavior. Women who self-identify as lesbian or WSW may have had, or continue to have, sexual contact with male partners.[29,36–39] This possibility is especially true for ethnic minority lesbian women, who reported more sexual contacts with men.[36] Further, ethnic minority women who identify as lesbian or bisexual may not report their sexual orientation and behaviors to health care providers as frequently as white lesbian women.[36] Therein lies a vulnerable trajectory of risk for minority lesbian women and minority WSW: lower perceptions of risk of STI, higher number of sexual contacts with male partners, nondisclosure of sexual risk behaviors to health care providers, and less access to minority community-based support networks. Bridges and colleagues[40] noted that African American women may lose community social and economic support if they identify as lesbian. There is a theoretic connection between social support and preventive health screenings.[41] Despite the potential importance of community support structures to health behavior, there is a paucity of community-based STI prevention initiatives for lesbian, bisexual, and WSW women.[42] To address this, Logie and colleagues[43] designed and piloted the Queer Women Conversations (QWC) study. QWC specifically tailored group-based educational components to a diverse range of WSW (lesbians, bisexual, queer, other WSW). At the 6-week mark after intervention, sexual risk practices, barrier use self-efficacy, STI knowledge, and sexual stigma were significantly affected. Although long-term results[43] were not sustained in the pilot for all outcomes, the pilot does provide an exploratory framework for further investigation about the role of community support and community connectedness[44] in addressing disparities in STI infection for this vulnerable population of women.

DISPARITIES IN UNMET MEDICAL NEEDS BY SEXUAL ORIENTATION
Health Care Access

There are multiple barriers to care at both the structural and individual level for sexual minority women.[45] Lack of health insurance coverage in addition to nonrecognition of same-sex partnerships was a major barrier that prevented many sexual minority women from obtaining employer-sponsored health insurance coverage through their partners.[46] In addition, sexual minority women are more likely to lack health insurance.[47–49] Another structural barrier is the lack of culturally competent providers trained in the health care needs of the LGBT community.[45,50–52] As a result, encounters with the health care environment are often negative because of perceived or internalized stigma. As such, several studies show that sexual minority women are more likely to delay health care and less likely to have a usual place of care.[47,48,53]

Preventive Health Care Services

Data show that lesbians are at increased risk for not receiving important preventive health services such as Pap smears and mammograms.[54–58] Extant literature shows that sexual minority women underuse cervical cancer screening services. Screening rates are estimated to be between 43% and 71%, compared with 73% in the general female population.[25,59–62] In addition to the risk factors identified among heterosexual women that contribute to nonreceipt of preventive health services, such as age, income, education, health insurance, and having a regular health care provider or site of care, sexual minority women may have additional risk factors. Sexual minority women may be hesitant to disclose their sexual orientation to a health care provider, for fear of discrimination,[63] physician ignorance regarding lesbian health issues caused by heteronormative health care services and providers, and lack of insurance coverage or access to partner benefits.[62,64] Bjorkman and Materud[65] highlight the unique challenges sexual minority women face in seeking health care, even though they experience some health problems more frequently than their heterosexual peers, caused by marginalization. This marginalization, which occurs when a person exists between 2 cultures but does not entirely feel connected to either, may result in feelings of isolation, low self-esteem, and predisposition to emotional stress. Discrimination experiences include heterosexual assumption, inappropriate questioning, and refusal of services.

Although there has been some work to identify factors that influence screening behaviors, more knowledge on factors unique to sexual minority women may assist with the development of tailored strategies to increase screening rates. As with heterosexual women, there seem to be age differences in gynecologic screening rates among sexual minority women. One study[62] found that the highest rates of gynecologic cancer screening among lesbians occurred in those 50 years old and older. The factors associated with the increased rates among older lesbians are unknown but may be caused by more consistent messaging. This nonparticipation in preventive health screenings is detrimental to the health of sexual minority women. Lack of screening may result in later detection and treatment of gynecologic cancers. Breast cancer risk assessment is particularly important because sexual minority women seem to have a higher risk for developing breast cancer compared with heterosexual women because of higher prevalence of nulliparity, older age at first live birth,[66] and obesity.[67]

INTERVENTIONS

There is little in the literature regarding interventions to address LGBT health disparities because this work is still in the early stages of development. However, sexual

Box 2	
Heterosexism and homophobia	
Term	**Definition**
Heterosexism	The belief that heterosexuality is a superior orientation, and failure to value alternative sexual identities
Homophobia	An irrational fear, prejudice, and hatred of gay individuals

Data from Chesir-Teran D, Hughes D. Heterosexism in high school and victimization among lesbian, gay, bisexual, and questioning students. J Youth Adolesc 2009;38(7):963–75; and Weinberg G. Society and the healthy homosexual. New York: St. Martens Press; 1972.

minority women report using certain strategies, such as screening and crusading, to address heterosexism and homophobia (defined in **Box 2**).[68,69]

Screening involves direct contact with a service provider, usually by phone, and asking questions about service philosophy. Providers are screened for their attitudes to the sexual orientation of potential clients. Any intimation of homophobia renders the service/provider homophobic. However, this may work in urban settings where there are lots of service provider options available.[70] This method may simply contribute to lack of engagement with health care providers, if there are few options and they are all found to be homophobic by the potential client. In addition, some sexual minorities report using a method called crusading. Crusading involves the potential client taking on the responsibility to educate and normalize their sexual orientation. They accept that some health care providers may not have had exposure to sexual minority women.

Although sexual minorities have an increased risk for substance abuse, intervention research with this particular subpopulation is sparse, and even more so among sexual minority women.[71] However, there is some evidence that sexual minorities, specifically men, prefer alternative treatments instead of mainstream forms of treatment.[72] At this point, it is not clear whether sexual minority women share this preference.

There is an obvious need for diversity training for health center staff and health care providers. The Gay and Lesbian Medical Association[73] produced *Guidelines for Care of Lesbian, Gay, Bisexual and Transgender Patients*, which should be used by primary care health care providers. The publication includes recommendations for staff sensitivity training and questions to include on LGBT-sensitive forms.

SUMMARY

Evolving shifts in policy resulting in greater inclusion of the LGBT community may have an impact on the health of sexual minority women. The inclusion of measures of sexual orientation, identity, and sexual behavior in population surveys has provided some insight into the health needs and health status of sexual minority women. However, it is imperative that clinicians understand the health needs of subgroups of sexual minority women, because there may be significant differences. Individual and community-based strategies that promote resilience and positive coping of minority stress among sexual minority women are areas in need of further investigation. In addition, additional efforts should be made to improve the disparities in health care access and use by targeting the health care providers and increasing cultural competency training.

REFERENCES

1. Ward BW, Dahlhamer JM, Galinsky AM, et al. Sexual orientation and health among U.S. adults: National Health Interview Survey, 2013. Natl Health Stat Report 2014;(77):1–10.

2. Institute of Medicine. The health of lesbian, gay, bisexual and transgender people: building a foundation for better understanding. Washington, DC: The National Academies Press; 2011.

3. Institute of Medicine. Lesbian health: current assessment and directions for the future. Washington, DC: The National Academies Press; 1999.

4. Simoni JM, Smith L, Oost KM, et al. Disparities in physical health conditions among lesbian and bisexual women: a systematic review of population-based studies. J Homosex 2016;13:1–13.

5. Gonzales G, Przedworski J, Henning-Smith C. Comparison of health and health risk factors between lesbian, gay, and bisexual adults and heterosexual adults in the United States: results from the National Health Interview Survey. JAMA Intern Med 2016;176(9):1344–51.

6. Meyer IH. Minority stress and mental health in gay men. J Health Soc Behav 1995;36(1):38–56.

7. Friedman RC. Homosexuality, psychopathology, and suicidality. Arch Gen Psychiatry 1999;56(10):887–8.

8. Meyer IH. Prejudice, social stress, and mental health in lesbian, gay, and bisexual populations: conceptual issues and research evidence. Psychol Bull 2003; 129(5):674–97.

9. Burton CM, Marshal MP, Chisolm DJ, et al. Sexual minority-related victimization as a mediator of mental health disparities in sexual minority youth: a longitudinal analysis. J Youth Adolesc 2013;42(3):394–402.

10. Marshal MP, Dietz LJ, Friedman MS, et al. Suicidality and depression disparities between sexual minority and heterosexual youth: a meta-analytic review. J Adolesc Health 2011;49(2):115–23.

11. Matthews AK, Hughes TL, Johnson T, et al. Prediction of depressive distress in a community sample of women: the role of sexual orientation. Am J Public Health 2002;92(7):1131–9.

12. King M, Semlyen J, Tai SS, et al. A systematic review of mental disorder, suicide, and deliberate self harm in lesbian, gay and bisexual people. BMC Psychiatry 2008;8:70.

13. Cochran SD, Mays VM, Sullivan JG. Prevalence of mental disorders, psychological distress, and mental health services use among lesbian, gay, and bisexual adults in the United States. J Consult Clin Psychol 2003;71(1):53–61.

14. Pakula B, Shoveller J, Ratner PA, et al. Prevalence and co-occurrence of heavy drinking and anxiety and mood disorders among gay, lesbian, bisexual, and heterosexual Canadians. Am J Public Health 2016;106(6):1042–8.

15. Everett BG, Talley AE, Hughes TL, et al. Sexual identity mobility and depressive symptoms: a longitudinal analysis of moderating factors among sexual minority women. Arch Sex Behav 2016;45(7):1731–44.

16. Mock SE, Eibach RP. Stability and change in sexual orientation identity over a 10-year period in adulthood. Arch Sex Behav 2012;41(3):641–8.

17. Ott MQ, Corliss HL, Wypij D, et al. Stability and change in self-reported sexual orientation identity in young people: application of mobility metrics. Arch Sex Behav 2011;40(3):519–32.

18. Savin-Williams RC, Joyner K, Rieger G. Prevalence and stability of self-reported sexual orientation identity during young adulthood. Arch Sex Behav 2012;41(1): 103–10.

19. Calzo JP, Antonucci TC, Mays VM, et al. Retrospective recall of sexual orientation identity development among gay, lesbian, and bisexual adults. Dev Psychol 2011;47(6):1658–73.

20. Flanders CE, Gibson MF, Goldberg AE, et al. Postpartum depression among visible and invisible sexual minority women: a pilot study. Arch Womens Ment Health 2016;19(2):299–305.

21. Gavin NI, Gaynes BN, Lohr KN, et al. Perinatal depression: a systematic review of prevalence and incidence. Obstet Gynecol 2005;106(5 Pt 1):1071–83.

22. Ross LE, Steele L, Goldfinger C, et al. Perinatal depressive symptomatology among lesbian and bisexual women. Arch Womens Ment Health 2007;10(2):53–9.

23. Trettin S, Moses-Kolko EL, Wisner KL. Lesbian perinatal depression and the heterosexism that affects knowledge about this minority population. Arch Womens Ment Health 2006;9(2):67–73.

24. Ross LE, Siegel A, Dobinson C, et al. "I don't want to turn totally invisible": mental health, stressors, and supports among bisexual women during the perinatal period. J GLBT Fam Stud 2012;8(2):137–54.

25. Kerr DL, Ding K, Thompson AJ. A comparison of lesbian, bisexual, and heterosexual female college undergraduate students on selected reproductive health screenings and sexual behaviors. Womens Health Issues 2013;23(6):e347–55.

26. Barbosa RM, Facchini R. Access to sexual health care for women who have sex with women in São Paulo, Brazil. Cad Saude Publica 2009;25(Suppl 2):S291–300 [in Portuguese].

27. Kuyper L, Vanwesenbeeck I. Examining sexual health differences between lesbian, gay, bisexual, and heterosexual adults: the role of sociodemographics, sexual behavior characteristics, and minority stress. J Sex Res 2011;48(2–3):263–74.

28. Bauer GR, Welles SL. Beyond assumptions of negligible risk: sexually transmitted diseases and women who have sex with women. Am J Public Health 2001;91(8):1282–6.

29. Marrazzo JM. Barriers to infectious disease care among lesbians. Emerg Infect Dis 2004;10(11):1974–8.

30. Power J, McNair R, Carr S. Absent sexual scripts: lesbian and bisexual women's knowledge, attitudes and action regarding safer sex and sexual health information. Cult Health Sex 2009;11(1):67–81.

31. McNair R. Risks and prevention of sexually transmissible infections among women who have sex with women. Sex Health 2005;2(4):209–17.

32. Dolan KA, Davis PW. Nuances and shifts in lesbian women's constructions of STI and HIV vulnerability. Soc Sci Med 2003;57(1):25–38.

33. Bailey JV, Farquhar C, Owen C, et al. Sexually transmitted infections in women who have sex with women. Sex Transm Infect 2004;80(3):244–6.

34. Chan SK, Thornton LR, Chronister KJ, et al. Likely female-to-female sexual transmission of HIV–Texas, 2012. MMWR Morb Mortal Wkly Rep 2014;63(10):209–12.

35. Marrazzo JM. Genital human papillomavirus infection in women who have sex with women: a concern for patients and providers. AIDS Patient Care STDS 2000;14(8):447–51.

36. Cochran SD, Mays VM. Disclosure of sexual preference to physicians by black lesbian and bisexual women. West J Med 1988;149(5):616–9.

37. Diamant AL, Schuster MA, McGuigan K, et al. Lesbians' sexual history with men: implications for taking a sexual history. Arch Intern Med 1999;159(22):2730–6.

38. Koh AS, Gomez CA, Shade S, et al. Sexual risk factors among self-identified lesbians, bisexual women, and heterosexual women accessing primary care settings. Sex Transm Dis 2005;32(9):563–9.

39. Muzny CA, Sunesara IR, Martin DH, et al. Sexually transmitted infections and risk behaviors among African American women who have sex with women: does sex with men make a difference? Sex Transm Dis 2011;38(12):1118–25.
40. Bridges SK, Selvidge MM, Matthews CR. Lesbian women of color: therapeutic issues and challenges. J Multicult Couns Devel 2003;31(2):113–31.
41. Glanz K, Rimer BK, Viswanath K, editors. Health behavior and health education: theory, research and practice. San Francisco (CA): John Wiley & Sons; 2008.
42. Logie CH, Navia D, Rwigema MJ, et al. A group-based HIV and sexually transmitted infections prevention intervention for lesbian, bisexual, queer and other women who have sex with women in Calgary and Toronto, Canada: study protocol for a non-randomised cohort pilot study. BMJ Open 2014;4(4):e005190.
43. Logie CH, Lacombe-Duncan A, Weaver J, et al. A pilot study of a group-based HIV and STI prevention intervention for lesbian, bisexual, queer, and other women who have sex with women in Canada. AIDS Patient Care STDS 2015;29(6):321–8.
44. Frost DM, Meyer IH. Measuring community connectedness among diverse sexual minority populations. J Sex Res 2012;49(1):36–49.
45. Dahlhamer JM, Galinsky AM, Joestl SS, et al. Barriers to health care among adults identifying as sexual minorities: a US National Study. Am J Public Health 2016;106(6):1116–22.
46. Ash MA, Badgett MV. Separate and unequal: the effect of unequal access to employment-based health insurance on same-sex and unmarried different-sex couples. Contemp Econ Policy 2006;24(4):582–99.
47. Heck JE, Sell RL, Gorin SS. Health care access among individuals involved in same-sex relationships. Am J Public Health 2006;96(6):1111–8.
48. Diamant AL, Wold C, Spritzer K, et al. Health behaviors, health status, and access to and use of health care: a population-based study of lesbian, bisexual, and heterosexual women. Arch Fam Med 2000;9(10):1043–51.
49. Bowen DJ, Bradford JB, Powers D, et al. Comparing women of differing sexual orientations using population-based sampling. Women Health 2004;40(3):19–34.
50. Alencar Albuquerque G, de Lima Garcia C, da Silva Quirino G, et al. Access to health services by lesbian, gay, bisexual, and transgender persons: systematic literature review. BMC Int Health Hum Rights 2016;16:2.
51. McNair RP, Hegarty K. Guidelines for the primary care of lesbian, gay, and bisexual people: a systematic review. Ann Fam Med 2010;8(6):533–41.
52. Li CC, Matthews AK, Aranda F, et al. Predictors and consequences of negative patient-provider interactions among a sample of African American sexual minority women. LGBT Health 2015;2(2):140–6.
53. Buchmueller T, Carpenter CS. Disparities in health insurance coverage, access, and outcomes for individuals in same-sex versus different-sex relationships, 2000-2007. Am J Public Health 2010;100(3):489–95.
54. Carroll NM. Optimal gynecologic and obstetric care for lesbians. Obstet Gynecol 1999;93(4):611–3.
55. Price JH, Easton AN, Telljohann SK, et al. Perceptions of cervical cancer and Pap smear screening behavior by women's sexual orientation. J Community Health 1996;21(2):89–105.
56. Roberts SJ, Sorensen L. Health related behaviors and cancer screening of lesbians: results from the Boston Lesbian Health Project. Women Health 1999; 28(4):1–12.
57. Diamant AL, Schuster MA, Lever J. Receipt of preventive health care services by lesbians. Am J Prev Med 2000;19(3):141–8.

58. Bazzi AR, Whorms DS, King DS, et al. Adherence to mammography screening guidelines among transgender persons and sexual minority women. Am J Public Health 2015;105(11):2356–8.

59. Charlton BM, Corliss HL, Missmer SA, et al. Reproductive health screening disparities and sexual orientation in a cohort study of U.S. adolescent and young adult females. J Adolesc Health 2011;49(5):505–10.

60. Agenor M, Krieger N, Austin SB, et al. Sexual orientation disparities in Papanicolaou test use among US women: the role of sexual and reproductive health services. Am J Public Health 2014;104(2):e68–73.

61. Fish J, Anthony D. UK National Lesbians and Health Care Survey. Women Health 2005;41(3):27–45.

62. Matthews AK, Brandenburg DL, Johnson TP, et al. Correlates of underutilization of gynecological cancer screening among lesbian and heterosexual women. Prev Med 2004;38(1):105–13.

63. Burgess D, Tran A, Lee R, et al. Effects of perceived discrimination on mental health and mental health services utilization among gay, lesbian, bisexual and transgender persons. J LGBT Health Res 2007;3(4):1–14.

64. Sabin JA, Riskind RG, Nosek BA. Health care providers' implicit and explicit attitudes toward lesbian women and gay men. Am J Public Health 2015;105(9): 1831–41.

65. Bjorkman M, Malterud K. Lesbian women's experiences with health care: a qualitative study. Scand J Prim Health Care 2009;27(4):238–43.

66. Meads C, Moore D. Breast cancer in lesbians and bisexual women: systematic review of incidence, prevalence and risk studies. BMC Public Health 2013;13: 1127.

67. Brandenburg DL, Matthews AK, Johnson TP, et al. Breast cancer risk and screening: a comparison of lesbian and heterosexual women. Women Health 2007;45(4):109–30.

68. Chesir-Teran D, Hughes D. Heterosexism in high school and victimization among lesbian, gay, bisexual, and questioning students. J Youth Adolesc 2009;38(7): 963–75.

69. Weinberg G. Society and the healthy homosexual. New York: St. Martens Press; 1972.

70. Hayman B, Wilkes L, Halcomb EJ, et al. Marginalised mothers: lesbian women negotiating heteronormative healthcare services. Contemp Nurse 2013;44(1): 120–7.

71. Green KE, Feinstein BA. Substance use in lesbian, gay, and bisexual populations: an update on empirical research and implications for treatment. Psychol Addict Behav 2012;26(2):265–78.

72. Dillworth TM, Kaysen D, Montoya HD, et al. Identification with mainstream culture and preference for alternative alcohol treatment approaches in a community sample. Behav Ther 2009;40(1):72–81.

73. Gay and Lesbian Medical Association. Guidelines for care of lesbian, gay, bisexual and transgender patients. Washington, DC: The Gay and Lesbian Medical Association; 2006.

Disparities in Fibroid Incidence, Prognosis, and Management

Shannon K. Laughlin-Tommaso, MD, MPH[a,b,*],
Vanessa L. Jacoby, MD, MAS[c], Evan R. Myers, MD, MPH[d]

KEYWORDS

- Fibroid • Leiomyoma • Race • Socioeconomic status • Rural • Disparity

KEY POINTS

- African American women have a greater burden of uterine fibroids, including higher prevalence, more severe disease, and worse treatment outcomes than white women.
- Access to fibroid treatment may be limited for women of lower socioeconomic status (SES) and rural location.
- The Comparing Options for Management: Patient-centered Results for Uterine Fibroids (COMPARE-UF) nationwide registry (www.compare-uf.org) partners with patients to understand these disparities and compare the effectiveness of fibroid treatments in different populations.

BACKGROUND

Fibroids, also called leiomyomas or myomas, are benign uterine tumors that develop from smooth muscle tissue and are present in up to 75% of women.[1] These tumors can cause heavy menstrual bleeding, pelvic pressure, and symptoms related to compression of the bowel and bladder; many may remain asymptomatic. The most common treatment of fibroids is hysterectomy, with approximately 200,000 cases

---

S.K. Laughlin-Tommaso: received research funding, paid to Mayo Clinic, from Truven Health Analytics Inc and from InSightec Ltd (Israel) for a focused ultrasonography ablation clinical trial; on the data safety monitoring board for the Uterine Leiomyoma (fibroid) Treatment With Radiofrequency Ablation (ULTRA) trial, Halt Medical, Inc). E.R. Myers: no conflicts relevant to fibroids. Consultant to Merck for human papillomavirus vaccines.
[a] Department of Obstetrics & Gynecology and Surgery, Mayo Clinic, 200 1st Street Southwest, Rochester, MN 55905, USA; [b] Department of Surgery, Mayo Clinic, 200 1st Street Southwest, Rochester, MN 55905, USA; [c] Department of Obstetrics, Gynecology, and Reproductive Sciences, University of California, San Francisco, 2356 Sutter Street, San Francisco, CA 94115, USA; [d] Department of Obstetrics & Gynecology, Duke Clinical Research Institute, Duke University, 2400 Pratt Street, Durham, NC 27705, USA
* Corresponding author. 200 1st Street Southwest, Rochester, MN 55905.
E-mail address: Laughlintommaso.shannon@mayo.edu

Obstet Gynecol Clin N Am 44 (2017) 81–94
http://dx.doi.org/10.1016/j.ogc.2016.11.007
0889-8545/17/© 2016 Elsevier Inc. All rights reserved.

annually in the United States.[2] For decades, hysterectomy was the only option for women who had completed childbearing. Many women now seek more minimally invasive treatment than hysterectomy. Unfortunately, minimally invasive options may not be accessible uniformly across all patient populations. The COMPARE-UF study is a multisite national registry with a goal of understanding the comparative effectiveness of treatment options and outcomes in a diverse population of premenopausal women with fibroids. This article discusses the racial and ethnic disparities in fibroid incidence, disease severity and progression, access to fibroid therapy, and surgical outcomes as well as the goal of the COMPARE-UF study to enroll a racially and ethnically diverse patient population.

Health disparities can be defined in many ways but, refer to differences that "systematically and negatively impact less advantaged groups."[3] Fibroids, like many other diseases, are subject to disparities between race/ethnic groups, SES, and access-to-care issues, such as insurance status and urban-centered treatment sites. How these disparities have an impact on underserved women and how the COMPARE-UF study is overcoming these obstacles are discussed.

RACIAL AND ETHNIC DISPARITIES

Racial and ethnic differences in prevalence, prognosis, and treatment options are prominent in fibroids. Nearly all of the data compare African American women with white women, due to scarce data on prevalence and treatment differences in Latina and Asian women. African American women are substantially more impacted by fibroids than women of other races and ethnicities. Fibroids are 2 to 3 times more common among African American women than white women. African American women develop fibroids at an earlier age, have more and larger tumors on diagnosis, have continued high rates of growth until menopause, and are more at risk for having surgical procedures. Despite this, African American women comprise only 15% of women in fibroid studies.[4]

Prevalence

Almost all studies have demonstrated a higher fibroid prevalence among African American women compared with white women. African American women have 2 to 3 times the risk of uterine fibroids based on ultrasound screening studies, prospective studies of clinically diagnosed fibroids, and pathologic studies of hysterectomy samples.[1,5–8] Although most of the prevalence data by race are from the United States, estimates from South Africa indicate similar differences between black and nonblack women.[9]

In the Nurses' Health Study, Hispanic and Asian women had similar prevalence of fibroids to white women.[7] Prevalence was similar for Hispanic and white women in a pregnant population as well.[6] Data are limited for Hispanic and Asian women.

Earlier Onset

Clinically significant fibroids develop 5 years earlier on average for African American women than white women.[1,8,10] Based on ultrasound screening studies of asymptomatic women, a substantial proportion of African American women develop fibroids in their early 20s.[5,6] Estimates for women 18 to 30 years old were 26% for black women and 7% for white women.[5] Among pregnant patients over 18 years, prevalence in an ultrasound screening study overall was 18% for African American women, 8% for white women, and 10% for Hispanic women and increased with age.[6] These differences were confirmed in older women in the Uterine Fibroid Study, where cumulative incidence was 80% for African American and 70% for white women by age 50.[1]

In a retrospective study of hysterectomy specimens, African American and Hispanic women tended to have surgery at a younger age than white and Asian women.[11]

Disease Severity

Not only do fibroids develop earlier in African American women but also disease severity tends to be worse than in white women. Fibroids are larger and more numerous in African American women in ultrasound screening trials.[1,6] At the time of treatment, African American women often have more fibroids, but total fibroid volume does not significantly differ.[12,13] In hysterectomy samples, uterine weight was found to be 100 g heavier in African American women than white women on average and more likely to contain 7 or more fibroids.[8] Hispanic women had similar fibroid size to African American women in an ultrasound screening study.[6]

Larger size has implications for treatment. In a longitudinal study, size of the largest fibroid was predictive of undergoing surgery.[14] Members of a large urban health plan were screened for fibroids and then recontacted 8 years later. The risk of a major uterine procedure increased with increasing size of the largest fibroid at baseline. For women with a baseline fibroid size greater than 4 cm, the risk of a uterine procedure increased 27-fold; this risk did not differ by race, but twice the number of African American versus white women were found to have large fibroids at baseline.[14]

There are many theories as to the higher risk and more severe disease in African American women (**Box 1**); however, the racial disparity in pathogenesis remains unexplained.[15–20]

Symptom Severity

African American women are at higher risk for more or worse symptoms than women of other racial and ethnic backgrounds. Studies have found that African American women were more likely to be anemic and have greater pelvic pain than white women.[8] In the Finding Genes for Fibroids study, 91% of African American women

---

Box 1
Fibroid risk factors that may vary between racial and ethnic groups

- Genetic variations
  - Unique gene polymorphisms leading to higher estrogen
  - Micro-RNA aberrant expression
  - Retinoic acid receptor expression
  - Aromatase levels

- Lifestyle factors
  - Diet
  - Body mass index
  - Smoking
  - Alcohol use
  - Physical activity
  - Diabetes mellitus
  - High blood pressure

- Environmental exposures
  - Vitamin D deficiency
  - Bisphenol A exposure
  - Psychosocial stressors

met severe symptom criteria compared with 71% of white women.[10] The criteria for severe symptoms included

- Heavy or prolonged menstrual bleeding
- Diagnosis before age 40
- Multiple surgeries for fibroids
- Hysterectomy for fibroids

Even after adjusting for known risk factors, such as body mass index, smoking, oral contraceptive pill use prior to age 20, age of menarche, parity, and red meat and alcohol consumption, race was still significantly associated with higher severity of fibroid disease.[10]

In a national Internet-based survey, 268 African American and 573 white women with fibroids responded. African American women had heavier or more prolonged menses (relative risk [RR] 1.51; 95% CI 1.05–2.18) and higher risk of anemia (RR 2.73; 95% CI 1.47–5.09) in multivariable models.[21] Abdominal pressure and pain, increased girth, passing clots, and fatigue were all significantly higher in African American women compared with white women. Family relationships and employment impacted by fibroids were a concern for all women, with slightly higher reporting in African American women.

Fibroid Growth and Regression

Because fibroids can be asymptomatic for much of the early stages of development, the rate of growth has been minimally studied. In the Fibroid Growth Study, median growth rates between African American women and white women were similar (12% and 10%, respectively). Fibroids from African American women, however, grew at a faster rate after age 45 than from white women (15% v. 2%).[22] In white women, age was related to a decline in growth rate for tumors but this was not true for African American women (**Fig. 1**).[22]

Parity is associated with a reduction in fibroid development, and one theory is that pregnancy and delivery actively degrade fibroid tissue. In a study of fibroid regression after pregnancy, African American women had less fibroid regression compared with white women (odds ratio [OR] 0.47; 95% CI, 0.25–0.88). Although African American women have larger fibroids, fibroid size was not associated with regression.[23]

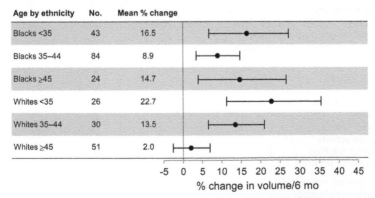

Fig. 1. Fibroid growth rate by race and age. (*Adapted from* Peddada SD, Laughlin SK, Miner K, et al. Growth of uterine leiomyomata among premenopausal black and white women. Proc Natl Acad Sci U S A 2008;105(50):19889.)

Treatment Differences

African American women are more likely to have
- Hysterectomy or myomectomy compared with a nonsurgical therapy
- Abdominal surgery instead of laparoscopic
- Complications or poor outcomes from surgery

Studies of women who undergo surgery for fibroids are critical for understanding the disparities in surgical burden. African American women have higher hysterectomy rates than white women in the United States in several studies. In a nationwide analysis, the rate of hysterectomy for fibroids was 37.6 per 10,000 black women compared with 16.4 per 10,000 white women.[24] In a California-based study, both African American women and Latina women had a higher risk of undergoing fibroid-related surgery, including hysterectomy and myomectomy, than non-Latina white women (RR 2.3 and 1.3, respectively).[25] In a 2007 Nationwide Inpatient Sample (NIS) study, African American women had 2.4 times the risk of hysterectomy and 6.8 times the risk of myomectomy compared with white women.[26] Pathologic studies have also confirmed this higher risk.[8,27]

Young African American women, in particular, are at risk for surgery that may affect future fertility. In a US insurance database study that examined patient characteristics that led to various fibroid-related treatments, there was an interaction between age and race (identified by racial density within a geographic location) that influenced procedure. A higher percentage of African American women in a region increased the chance of a uterine-sparing procedure over hysterectomy.[28] This was strongest in women aged 18 to 34 years but still present in women aged 45 to 54. Because African American women experience fibroid symptoms at a younger age, uterine conservation is paramount for fertility preservation. Among the uterine-sparing techniques, the regions with the highest density of African American residents were less likely to undergo endometrial ablation, a minor surgery that is not compatible with future childbearing, compared with myomectomy.[28]

Selection of surgical approach also varies with race and ethnicity.[29] In a US population-based study of hysterectomy for abnormal uterine bleeding or fibroids, African American and Hispanic women were 56% and 42%, respectively, less likely to undergo a laparoscopic hysterectomy compared with an abdominal hysterectomy.[30] This remained true even when adjusted for the presence of leiomyomas, which may make minimally invasive surgery more difficult; however, investigators were unable to control for uterine size or number of fibroids. The racial differences in uterine fibroid size at presentation may play a role in choice of surgical approach. In a 2005 NIS study, 62% of abdominal hysterectomies were for uterine fibroids[31]; African American, Latina, and Asian women all had 40% to 50% lower odds of laparoscopic hysterectomy compared with white women. Similar results were found using the 2009 NIS[29]; however, this sampling found that Native American women had a higher chance of laparoscopic hysterectomy than white women. Although the presence of fibroids did influence surgical route, having fibroids did not account for the total difference in race; medically underserved women may be excluded from technologically advanced surgeries.[31] The rate of increase in laparoscopic hysterectomy is higher for white women than black or Hispanic women, indicating a growing disparity in minimally invasive surgery in the future (**Fig. 2**).[32]

Hysterectomy and myomectomy can be performed in either an inpatient hospital setting or an ambulatory setting. Hospital costs are higher and length of stay is longer for inpatient surgery. Black and Hispanic women had higher rates of inpatient surgery (60%–70%) compared with white women (40%–46%) in the 13-state Healthcare Cost and Utilization Project.[33]

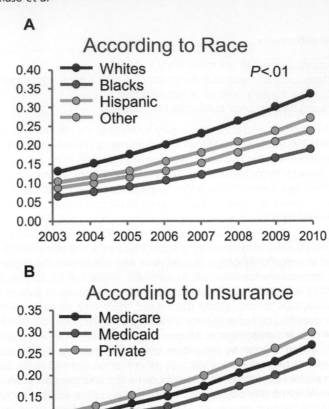

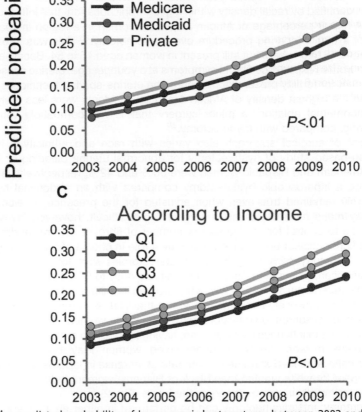

Fig. 2. The predicted probability of laparoscopic hysterectomy between 2003 and 2010 according to (*A*) Race, (*B*) Insurance status, and (*C*) Quartile (Q) of income, with Q4 the most affluent. (*Adapted from* Lee J, Jennings K, Borahay MA, et al. Trends in the national distribution of laparoscopic hysterectomies from 2003 to 2010. J Minim Invasive Gynecol 2014;21(4):659.)

There is regional variation for hysterectomy in the United States. The South has a higher incidence of hysterectomy than Northeast, Midwest, or West[31]; compared with the Northeast, women in the South have approximately half the chance of having a uterine-sparing procedure than having a hysterectomy.[28] The South also has the highest percentage of reproductive age African American women. The relative contributions of clinical factors, such as more severe symptoms or larger fibroids, in African American women or social factors, such as clinician experience and preference, patient preference, or family or community experience with hysterectomy, to these regional differences is unclear.

As discussed previously, a major limitation of all of these population-based studies is that factors that may contribute to choice of treatment or surgical approach, such as uterine size, number and location of fibroids, obesity, or prior surgical history, are not captured in administrative data.[34]

Surgical Outcomes

In addition to carrying a higher burden of surgery, African American women are more at risk for poor surgical outcomes. Hysterectomy complications, in-hospital mortality, and length of stay were higher in African American than white women.[35] Some of this variation may be related to the higher rate of abdominal hysterectomy among African American women.[31] Additionally, African American women have larger uteri or more fibroids, which increase the risk of complications, such as cuff cellulitis and transfusion.[8,36,37] When uterine size, number of fibroids, and presence of comorbidities were controlled, race was not significantly associated with higher complications; however, uterine size and number of fibroids increased the risk approximately 85% and the risk of transfusion 6-fold and 2-fold, respectively.[37]

In a California-based study, Asian women were also more at risk for hysterectomy complications than white women, even with adjustment for age, indications, other comorbidities, and surgeries.[38] Hispanic women had lower risk of complications for vaginal and abdominal hysterectomy but an 11% increase in risk for subtotal hysterectomy compared with white women.

Nonsurgical therapy for fibroids may have less disparity in outcomes by race, but evidence is limited. In a study of magnetic resonance–guided focused ultrasound ablation, African American women had similar outcomes to non–African American women despite higher total fibroid number and younger age.[13]

Reproductive Outcomes

Pregnancy outcomes differ by race and ethnicity as well. Fibroids are associated with higher rates of miscarriage, cesarean section, preterm birth and low birth weight, and intrauterine fetal death,[39,40] although some of the observed associations may be due to issues, such as detection bias (for example, incidental fibroids noted at the time of imaging and/or cesarean section because of pregnancy complications and subsequently noted on discharge data). Because African American women develop fibroids at a young age, they may be at greater risk for fibroid-related reproductive complications than white women. Some studies have found that fibroids, in particular those that abut or distort the endometrium, are associated with increased rates of infertility. Therefore, the higher incidence of fibroids among African American women may manifest in increased infertility rates.

In addition to the impacts on fertility and pregnancy, infertility services may be less accessible. Low-income women and women with less than 12 years of education are the least likely to access fertility services; women of racial minorities are overrepresented in these groups in the United States and, thus, do not seek fertility services as frequently.[41] In a military population that provided equal access to care to all women, racial minorities were represented in fertility clinics similarly to the racial distribution of the US population, indicating that there are similar fertility needs but less access to fertility services in the general US population.[41] In this study, clinical and live birth rates, implantation rates, and spontaneous abortion rates were all negatively affected by the presence of fibroids.[41] Because African American women were 3 times as likely to have fibroids, adverse fertility outcomes were more common among African American women, with an increased rate of spontaneous abortion rate reaching statistical significance.[41]

COMPARING OPTIONS FOR MANAGEMENT: PATIENT-CENTERED RESULTS FOR UTERINE FIBROIDS IS ADDRESSING DISPARITIES

As discussed previously, currently available population-based data sources on disparities in choice of fibroid treatments and outcomes of treatment among African American women compared with white women do not provide relevant information on clinical factors that may contribute to treatment choice and outcome. The inability to adjust for the known racial differences in these clinical factors prevents drawing inferences about the contribution of other nonclinical factors on disparities in treatment choice and outcome.

The COMPARE-UF registry, a large national prospective observational study of women undergoing treatment of uterine fibroids, is collecting detailed data on pretreatment uterine and fibroid anatomy and relevant medical and surgical history as well as treatment details and pretreatment and post-treatment outcomes. The aim of the study is to compare the effectiveness of fibroid treatment in different populations and the subsequent effect on reproduction. The focus of the outcomes is patient centered, including symptom relief, quality of life, complications, and reproductive outcomes. COMPARE-UF allows women to enroll, consent, and complete all study questionnaires online; this approach supports participation and follow-up for rural populations that may be remote from clinical centers. Approximately 50% of the expected participants will be African American women (**Fig. 3**),

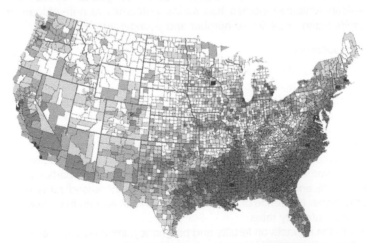

Fig. 3. Map of the United States showing the locations of COMPARE-UF enrollment centers (symbols). Shaded areas indicate the distribution of African American women 15 to 44 years old in each county based on 2010 census data.

allowing the registry to specifically address the impact of disparities in fibroid severity on treatment choice and outcomes. One unique aspect of COMPARE-UF is the extensive degree of patient involvement in identifying and prioritizing research questions, especially which outcomes to measure, governance of the registry, and engagement with the broader community to encourage participation and, ultimately, disseminate research findings.

DISPARITIES RELATED TO SOCIOECONOMIC STATUS
Fibroid Prevalence

Psychosocial stress has been associated with a higher risk of fibroids in several studies; there is a dose-response relationship, where the higher number of major life events and stress intensity increased the risk of fibroids.[42,43] Inability to meet basic needs and having an inadequate income have been shown to affect stress levels and subsequent health.[44,45] Women tend to be paid less and have fewer work benefits than men. In addition, one-quarter of women with fibroids have reported that symptoms have kept them from reaching potential at work and have limited work-related activities.[46]

In the National Institute of Environmental Health Sciences Sister Study, childhood socioeconomic markers, including highest level of education for the household, being poor, and not having enough time to eat, were associated with the incidence of fibroids.[47] There was a 24% increase in fibroids by age 35 with reports of being poor as a child (RR 1.24; 95% CI, 0.99–1.55) and a 28% increase if 2 or more of the factors were reported (RR 1.28; 95% CI, 1.01–1.63).

Treatment Differences

Fibroid treatment is affected by SES in many studies. Hysterectomy rates are higher among women in lower SES brackets. In a study in Rome, women in the least affluent level had a 34% higher risk of hysterectomy than those in the most affluent level, with a significant trend across SES.[48] Women ages 35 to 49 years in the least affluent group had a 60% higher risk of hysterectomy, a majority of which were for fibroids, than women of the same age in the most affluent group. The investigators were unable to determine the prevalence of disease within each SES level; however, risk factors for fibroids, such as low parity and hormone replacement therapy, have been associated with higher affluence.

Similar findings were seen in a Danish population-based cohort and in US women, where hysterectomy rates were attributed to women of lower SES not seeking care until later stages of disease.[49,50] When hysterectomy by fibroid indication was evaluated in the United States, however, neither educational level nor SES status was associated with risk.[51] Using a US insurance database, Borah and colleagues[28] found that increasing income and education levels was associated with using a uterine-sparing procedure (myomectomy, endometrial ablation, or uterine artery embolization) over hysterectomy.

- Laparoscopic surgery is less common in women with Medicaid than laparotomy.

Income and insurance status influences the type of hysterectomy performed.[31,52,53] In a US-based study from 2005, women with household incomes lower than $61,000 and women without private health insurance were less likely to undergo laparoscopy than abdominal surgery, irrespective of race or ethnicity.[31] This was confirmed in a population-based study of hysterectomies for abnormal uterine bleeding or fibroids in the United States. Women in higher income brackets were 12% to 18% more likely to have a laparoscopy than laparotomy. Those with private insurance were 50% more likely to receive a laparoscopic hysterectomy over an abdominal hysterectomy compared with women on Medicaid.[30] In a US NIS from 2009, Medicaid and self-pay patients were 20% to 30% less likely to have a laparoscopic hysterectomy than a laparotomy.[29] Lower health literacy or limited access to hospitals with better technology may contribute to these differences; however, because private insurance reimburses physicians at a higher amount, there is a financial disincentive to offer a more expensive minimally invasive procedure to women with Medicare or Medicaid.[31] Even in women with uterine cancer, income, race, and insurance status influence the type of hysterectomy after adjustment for the presence of fibroids.[52]

- Although the number of laparoscopic surgeries has increased, the difference in rates according to income has stayed stable[32] (see **Fig. 2**).

Inpatient surgery in general is more common among women with Medicaid or no insurance compared with women with private insurance.

Reproductive Outcomes

In the Coronary Artery Risk Development in Young Adults women's study, SES played a significant role in infertility for black women but less so for white women.[54] Ever-infertile women were more likely to have a lower income, lower education, and difficulty paying for basics. When analyses were adjusted, age and hormonal contraception use, race, lower education, and presence of fibroids still increased the risk of infertility.

RURAL/URBAN

Access to fibroid therapy other than hysterectomy is limited mainly to urban areas (**Fig. 4**). Many of the newer less-invasive therapies are studied at major universities in highly populated areas.

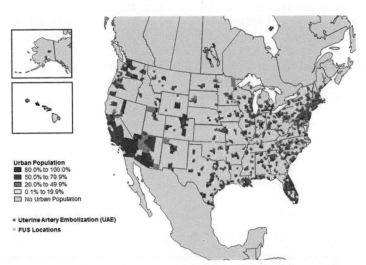

Fig. 4. Map of the United States demonstrating the locations of magnetic resonance–guided focused ultrasound ablation surgery (FUS) (Green dot) and uterine artery embolization (Pink dot). The size of the symbol represents the approximate number of available centers in a region providing these fibroid therapies. (*Courtesy of* the Mayo Foundation for Medical Education and Research, Rochester MN; with permission.)

Rural/urban setting may not influence surgical therapies as much as other sociodemographic factors. In the 2005 NIS, rural versus urban hospital setting was not associated with surgical approach when comparing laparoscopic with abdominal surgery.[31] In the 2009 NIS, where urban/rural location was subdivided into 6 population-based categories, location was not associated with surgical approach.[29] The NIS is limited, however, to inpatient procedures; geographic disparities in the availability of rural outpatient surgical centers may overestimate the rate of laparoscopic procedures in the NIS because these are performed as an inpatient procedure.

By contrast, a Vancouver, Canada, study found that rural residence (<10,000 inhabitants in a postal code) increased the chance of undergoing a laparoscopic hysterectomy by 90% even when fibroid indication was taken into account. Having the surgery done at an urban location, however, was associated with a 22-fold increase in laparoscopic surgery (adjusted OR 22.2; 95% CI, 2.3–192.3).

THE INTERPLAY OF DISPARITIES

The evidence discussed previously demonstrates substantial disparities in treatment choice and outcomes based on race/ethnicity, insurance status, and urban/rural location. In practice, there is likely to be significant overlap across these domains—African American women will be less likely to have private insurance in many locations,[55] and there may be substantial differences by race and insurance status within a given metropolitan area or in rural areas in different states. The implementation of the Affordable Care Act (ACA) has led to significant improvements in insurance status and access to care, but significant disparities persist, particularly in states that have not participated in Medicaid expansion.[56] Comparing changes in fibroid treatment choice and outcomes by race, insurance status, and rural/urban location in the context of ACA implementation provides an opportunity to gain more insight into these disparities, particularly if integrated with data from studies, such as COMPARE-UF, which will provide complementary data on detailed clinical factors.

SUMMARY

Disparities in access to a diverse range of fibroid treatment options can have a significant impact on quality of life and morbidity in the care of women with fibroids. There is still much to learn about the roles that race, ethnicity, SES, and geographic location play in treatment options. Implementation of the ACA will provide broader treatment options to all women, and the first nationwide fibroid registry, COMPARE-UF, will allow better understanding of choices made when health care access is extended.

REFERENCES

1. Day Baird D, Dunson DB, Hill MC, et al. High cumulative incidence of uterine leiomyoma in black and white women: ultrasound evidence. Am J Obstet Gynecol 2003;188(1):100–7.

2. Wu JM, Wechter ME, Geller EJ, et al. Hysterectomy rates in the United States, 2003. Obstet Gynecol 2007;110(5):1091–5.

3. Dehlendorf C, Bryant AS, Huddleston HG, et al. Health disparities: definitions and measurements. Am J Obstet Gynecol 2010;202(3):212–3.

4. Taran FA, Brown HL, Stewart EA. Racial diversity in uterine leiomyoma clinical studies. Fertil Steril 2010;94(4):1500–3.

5. Marsh EE, Ekpo GE, Cardozo ER, et al. Racial differences in fibroid prevalence and ultrasound findings in asymptomatic young women (18-30 years old): a pilot study. Fertil Steril 2013;99(7):1951–7.

6. Laughlin SK, Baird DD, Savitz DA, et al. Prevalence of uterine leiomyomas in the first trimester of pregnancy: an ultrasound-screening study. Obstet Gynecol 2009;113(3):630–5.

7. Marshall LM, Spiegelman D, Barbieri RL, et al. Variation in the incidence of uterine leiomyoma among premenopausal women by age and race. Obstet Gynecol 1997;90(6):967–73.

8. Kjerulff KH, Langenberg P, Seidman JD, et al. Uterine leiomyomas. Racial differences in severity, symptoms and age at diagnosis. J Reprod Med 1996;41(7):483–90.

9. Butt JL, Jeffery ST, Van der Spuy ZM. An audit of indications and complications associated with elective hysterectomy at a public service hospital in South Africa. Int J Gynaecol Obstet 2012;116(2):112–6.

10. Huyck KL, Panhuysen CI, Cuenco KT, et al. The impact of race as a risk factor for symptom severity and age at diagnosis of uterine leiomyomata among affected sisters. Am J Obstet Gynecol 2008;198(2):168.e1-9.

11. Wei JJ, Chiriboga L, Arslan AA, et al. Ethnic differences in expression of the dysregulated proteins in uterine leiomyomata. Hum Reprod 2006;21(1):57–67.

12. Pron G, Cohen M, Soucie J, et al. The Ontario Uterine Fibroid Embolization Trial. Part 1. Baseline patient characteristics, fibroid burden, and impact on life. Fertil Steril 2003;79(1):112–9.

13. Machtinger R, Fennessy FM, Stewart EA, et al. MR-guided focused ultrasound (MRgFUS) is effective for the distinct pattern of uterine fibroids seen in African-American women: data from phase III/IV, non-randomized, multicenter clinical trials. J Ther Ultrasound 2013;1:23.

14. Baird DD, Saldana TM, Shore DL, et al. A single baseline ultrasound assessment of fibroid presence and size is strongly predictive of future uterine procedure: 8-year follow-up of randomly sampled premenopausal women aged 35-49 years. Hum Reprod 2015;30(12):2936–44.

15. Wise LA, Laughlin-Tommaso SK. Epidemiology of uterine fibroids: from menarche to menopause. Clin Obstet Gynecol 2016;59(1):2–24.

16. Wise LA, Ruiz-Narvaez EA, Palmer JR, et al. African ancestry and genetic risk for uterine leiomyomata. Am J Epidemiol 2012;176(12):1159–68.

17. Wise LA, Palmer JR, Cozier YC, et al. Perceived racial discrimination and risk of uterine leiomyomata. Epidemiology 2007;18(6):747–57.

18. Ishikawa H, Reierstad S, Demura M, et al. High aromatase expression in uterine leiomyoma tissues of African-American women. J Clin Endocrinol Metab 2009;94(5):1752–6.

19. Baird DD, Hill MC, Schectman JM, et al. Vitamin d and the risk of uterine fibroids. Epidemiology 2013;24(3):447–53.

20. Catherino WH, Eltoukhi HM, Al-Hendy A. Racial and ethnic differences in the pathogenesis and clinical manifestations of uterine leiomyoma. Semin Reprod Med 2013;31(5):370–9.

21. Stewart EA, Nicholson WK, Bradley L, et al. The burden of uterine fibroids for African-American women: results of a national survey. J Womens Health (Larchmt) 2013;22(10):807–16.

22. Peddada SD, Laughlin SK, Miner K, et al. Growth of uterine leiomyomata among premenopausal black and white women. Proc Natl Acad Sci U S A 2008;105(50):19887–92.

23. Laughlin SK, Hartmann KE, Baird DD. Postpartum factors and natural fibroid regression. Am J Obstet Gynecol 2011;204(6):496.e1-6.
24. Wilcox LS, Koonin LM, Pokras R, et al. Hysterectomy in the United States, 1988-1990. Obstet Gynecol 1994;83(4):549–55.
25. Templeman C, Marshall SF, Clarke CA, et al. Risk factors for surgically removed fibroids in a large cohort of teachers. Fertil Steril 2009;92(4):1436–46.
26. Wechter ME, Stewart EA, Myers ER, et al. Leiomyoma-related hospitalization and surgery: prevalence and predicted growth based on population trends. Am J Obstet Gynecol 2011;205(5):492.e1-5.
27. Moore AB, Flake GP, Swartz CD, et al. Association of race, age and body mass index with gross pathology of uterine fibroids. J Reprod Med 2008;53(2):90–6.
28. Borah BJ, Laughlin-Tommaso SK, Myers ER, et al. Association Between Patient Characteristics and Treatment Procedure Among Patients With Uterine Leiomyomas. Obstet Gynecol 2016;127(1):67–77.
29. Cohen SL, Vitonis AF, Einarsson JI. Updated hysterectomy surveillance and factors associated with minimally invasive hysterectomy. JSLS 2014;18(3).
30. Abenhaim HA, Azziz R, Hu J, et al. Socioeconomic and racial predictors of undergoing laparoscopic hysterectomy for selected benign diseases: analysis of 341487 hysterectomies. J Minim Invasive Gynecol 2008;15(1):11–5.
31. Jacoby VL, Autry A, Jacobson G, et al. Nationwide use of laparoscopic hysterectomy compared with abdominal and vaginal approaches. Obstet Gynecol 2009;114(5):1041–8.
32. Lee J, Jennings K, Borahay MA, et al. Trends in the national distribution of laparoscopic hysterectomies from 2003 to 2010. J Minim Invasive Gynecol 2014;21(4):656–61.
33. Barrett ML, Weiss AJ, Stocks C, et al. Procedures to treat benign uterine fibroids in hospital inpatient and hospital-based ambulatory surgery settings, 2013: statistical brief #200. Rockville (MD): Healthcare Cost and Utilization Project (HCUP) Statistical Briefs; 2006.
34. Myers ER, Steege JF. Risk adjustment for complications of hysterectomy: limitations of routinely collected administrative data. Am J Obstet Gynecol 1999;181(3):567–75.
35. Kjerulff KH, Guzinski GM, Langenberg PW, et al. Hysterectomy and race. Obstet Gynecol 1993;82(5):757–64.
36. Hillis SD, Marchbanks PA, Peterson HB. Uterine size and risk of complications among women undergoing abdominal hysterectomy for leiomyomas. Obstet Gynecol 1996;87(4):539–43.
37. Roth TM, Gustilo-Ashby T, Barber MD, et al. Effects of race and clinical factors on short-term outcomes of abdominal myomectomy. Obstet Gynecol 2003;101(5 Pt 1):881–4.
38. Smith LH, Waetjen LE, Paik CK, et al. Trends in the safety of inpatient hysterectomy for benign conditions in California, 1991-2004. Obstet Gynecol 2008;112(3):553–61.
39. Pritts EA, Parker WH, Olive DL. Fibroids and infertility: an updated systematic review of the evidence. Fertil Steril 2009;91(4):1215–23.
40. Lai J, Caughey AB, Qidwai GI, et al. Neonatal outcomes in women with sonographically identified uterine leiomyomata. J Matern Fetal Neonatal Med 2012;25(6):710–3.
41. Feinberg EC, Larsen FW, Catherino WH, et al. Comparison of assisted reproductive technology utilization and outcomes between Caucasian and African American patients in an equal-access-to-care setting. Fertil Steril 2006;85(4):888–94.

42. Vines AI, Ta M, Esserman DA. The association between self-reported major life events and the presence of uterine fibroids. Womens Health Issues 2010;20(4): 294–8.
43. Boynton-Jarrett R, Rich-Edwards JW, Jun HJ, et al. Abuse in childhood and risk of uterine leiomyoma: the role of emotional support in biologic resilience. Epidemiology 2011;22(1):6–14.
44. Williams D, Lawler KA. Stress and illness in low-income women: the roles of hardiness, John Henryism, and race. Women Health 2001;32(4):61–75.
45. Schulz A, Israel B, Williams D, et al. Social inequalities, stressors and self reported health status among African American and white women in the Detroit metropolitan area. Soc Sci Med 2000;51(11):1639–53.
46. Borah BJ, Nicholson WK, Bradley L, et al. The impact of uterine leiomyomas: a national survey of affected women. Am J Obstet Gynecol 2013;209(4):319.e1-20.
47. D'Aloisio AA, Baird DD, DeRoo LA, et al. Association of intrauterine and early-life exposures with diagnosis of uterine leiomyomata by 35 years of age in the Sister Study. Environ Health Perspect 2010;118(3):375–81.
48. Materia E, Rossi L, Spadea T, et al. Hysterectomy and socioeconomic position in Rome, Italy. J Epidemiol Community Health 2002;56(6):461–5.
49. Kjerulff K, Langenberg P, Guzinski G. The socioeconomic correlates of hysterectomies in the United States. Am J Public Health 1993;83(1):106–8.
50. Settnes A, Jorgensen T. Hysterectomy in a Danish cohort. Prevalence, incidence and socio-demographic characteristics. Acta Obstet Gynecol Scand 1996;75(3): 274–80.
51. Brett KM, Marsh JV, Madans JH. Epidemiology of hysterectomy in the United States: demographic and reproductive factors in a nationally representative sample. J Womens Health 1997;6(3):309–16.
52. Esselen KM, Vitonis A, Einarsson J, et al. Health Care disparities in hysterectomy for gynecologic cancers: data from the 2012 National Inpatient Sample. Obstet Gynecol 2015;126(5):1029–39.
53. Luoto R, Hemminki E, Topo P, et al. Hysterectomy among Finnish women: prevalence and women's own opinions. Scand J Soc Med 1992;20(4):209–12.
54. Wellons MF, Lewis CE, Schwartz SM, et al. Racial differences in self-reported infertility and risk factors for infertility in a cohort of black and white women: the CARDIA Women's Study. Fertil Steril 2008;90(5):1640–8.
55. Smith JC, Medalia C. U.S. Census bureau, current population reports, P60–253, health insurance coverage in the United States: 2014. Washington, DC: U.S. Government Printing Office; 2015. Available at: https://www.census.gov/content/dam/Census/library/publications/2015/demo/p60-253.pdf.
56. French MT, Homer J, Gumus G, et al. Key provisions of the patient protection and Affordable Care Act (ACA): a systematic review and presentation of early research findings. Health Serv Res 2016;51(5):1735–71.

Patient-centered Care to Address Barriers for Pregnant Women with Opioid Dependence

Mary Beth Sutter, MD[a],*, Sarah Gopman, MD[a],
Lawrence Leeman, MD, MPH[a],[b]

KEYWORDS

- Perinatal substance use • Incarceration • Harm reduction

KEY POINTS

- Many women with substance use disorders in pregnancy are underserved and delay obtaining prenatal care because of comorbidities of homelessness, poverty, mental health issues, social stigma regarding substance abuse in pregnancy, and a lack of adequate resources for substance abuse treatment.
- Punitive laws for substance-using pregnant women are unproductive and may discourage women from seeking care.
- Optimal care involves multidisciplinary cooperation between maternity care, substance abuse treatment, case management, and neonatal care teams.
- A family-centered model using harm reduction methods can improve outcomes for mothers and babies.

BACKGROUND AND EPIDEMIOLOGY

Women who use substances in pregnancy are an underserved population with a higher risk for maternal morbidity and neonatal morbidity and mortality. Maternal substance use affects all socioeconomic classes and the current opioid epidemic has brought heroin and prescription opioid addiction to many communities with minimal resources for treatment. Exposure to illicit substances in pregnancy increases the rates of preterm birth, placental abruption, intrauterine growth restriction, and other poor outcomes.[1] Infants affected by maternal substance use in pregnancy face

Disclosure: The authors have nothing to disclose.
[a] Department of Family and Community Medicine, University of New Mexico, MSC 09 5040, 1 University of New Mexico, Albuquerque, NM 87131, USA; [b] Department of Obstetrics and Gynecology, MSC 10 5580, 1 University of New Mexico, Albuquerque, NM 87131, USA
* Corresponding author.
E-mail address: msutter@salud.unm.edu

Obstet Gynecol Clin N Am 44 (2017) 95–107
http://dx.doi.org/10.1016/j.ogc.2016.11.004
0889-8545/17/© 2016 Elsevier Inc. All rights reserved.

obgyn.theclinics.com

challenges of withdrawal in the neonatal period as well as possible developmental effects persisting into childhood.

By self-report in 2013 to 2014, 5.3% of women aged 15 to 44 years were using illicit drugs during pregnancy.[2] Marijuana was the most common substance used at 4.1%, followed by nonmedical use of prescription drugs at 1.3%.[2] Substance use was more common in the first trimester at 8.9%, tapering to 5.3% in the second trimester and 1.9% in the third trimester.[2] Illicit drugs other than marijuana were used by 2% of pregnant women, including cocaine, heroin, hallucinogens, inhalants, and methamphetamines.[2]

These rates, based on self-report, are known to underestimate the proportion of the pregnant population with substance abuse issues. Many pregnant women do not disclose substance use because of concerns for confidentiality, stigmatization, removal of their children, incarceration, and other legal repercussions. Even in a prenatal program designed specifically for women with substance use problems, the sensitivity of self-reported drug use for all illicit substances was less than 60%.[3] Women may also disclose use, but report the timing of drug use inaccurately because of feelings of guilt regarding use in pregnancy. In another study, most women in a prenatal clinic for women with substance use issues with a positive urine drug screen reported recent drug use (78% marijuana, 86% cocaine); however, the most recent use report was often outside of the assay detection window (14% marijuana, 57% cocaine) indicating a trend toward reporting drug use as having occurred earlier in pregnancy.[4]

Illicit drug use in 2013 to 2014 among all women of reproductive age (15–44 years) is reported at 12.1%, which is up from 10.7% in 2011 to 2012.[2] The largest increase in use was seen in marijuana and nonmedical use of prescription opioids and stimulants.[2] Marijuana is increasingly legal and widely available. There has been a rapid increase in prescription opioid abuse over the last decade.[1,5] The demographic characteristics of pregnant women using illicit substances has also changed, necessitating that all obstetrician gynecologists, family physicians, and nurse midwives offering prenatal care have an understanding of how to screen and care for women with substance use disorders. Safe and responsible prescribing of opioid medications is the responsibility of all physicians holding a federal prescribing license.[6] Recent efforts to educate physicians regarding appropriate chronic use of opioids and the importance of checking prescription registries is decreasing the supply available from diversion, which may be increasing the transition of addicted women to heroin.[6,7] There is emerging evidence that women may progress more rapidly than men in the disease course of addiction and have a unique set of medical, psychiatric, and social considerations.[8] Pregnant women with substance abuse are a particularly vulnerable population.[9]

HOUSING, FOOD, AND TRANSPORTATION INSECURITY

Pregnant women struggling with substance use have many barriers to accessing resources, including housing, transportation, food, and job security. These social barriers are not necessarily tied to substance use itself, but rather the combination of low socioeconomic status and chaotic lifestyles.[10]

Housing stability is an important consideration and may affect maternal and infant safety and relapse rates. A disproportionate number of women struggling with substance use experience housing instability through all or part of pregnancy.[11] Others may have unsafe housing environments, including environments in which a partner or members of a social network are still abusing drugs, or in which domestic violence is occurring. Other women may have estranged friends and family during their struggle with substance use and have no options for social support. Inpatient treatment programs, which may be legally mandated, often do not allow children, requiring pregnant women to leave their existing children with their families, friends, or foster care, including in potentially unsafe environments.

Homelessness during pregnancy is an independent risk factor for adverse perinatal outcomes beyond lack of prenatal care and other socioeconomic factors.[12,13] Homeless women have 2.9 times increased likelihood of having a preterm birth, 6.9 times for birth weight less than 2000 g, and 3.3 times for a newborn small for gestational age.[11] When substance use coexists with homelessness these odds increase to 5.9 times for preterm birth, 16.6 times for birth weight less than 2000 g, and 5.6 times for a newborn small for gestational age.[11] Unstable housing, defined as living in more than 2 places during a pregnancy, is also associated with lack of prenatal care and with substance use during pregnancy.[10] The absolute risk associated with housing instability in pregnancy compares with preexisting diabetes and chronic hypertension and should therefore be considered a high-risk obstetric issue.[11]

Transportation is also a major barrier for pregnant substance-using women. They may lack a vehicle because of poverty, and may lack friends or family who own a vehicle and are sober. They may also encounter barriers to using public transportation, including cost, inability to register for subsidized fares because of illiteracy, lack of identification, lack of an address, or past legal actions. Insurance companies may provide transportation for medical visits during pregnancy, but often do not allow other children or partners to participate in the use of this transportation.

Enrolling in Medicaid can also be a challenge for pregnant women struggling with substance use. Navigation of the system can be difficult while coping with other stressors, facing a lack of transportation, and without necessary resources such as an identification card.

SOCIETAL STIGMA AND CRIMINALIZATION

There is a great deal of stigma facing pregnant women struggling with substance use from both the medical community and society at large. The stigma has persisted despite a greater understanding of addiction as a disease. In the 1980s the increasing rate of substance abuse in pregnancy was accompanied by the myth of so-called crack babies: infants who were developmentally compromised, unlikely to be able to perform at school and work, and at high risk for criminal activity. As a response, punitive approaches, including long-term incarceration, began to appear as a means to combat substance abuse.[14] Punitive approaches are sometimes applied not only to women using illicit substances but also to women on medication-assisted therapy (MAT), such as methadone or buprenorphine. These approaches can include arrest, detention, prosecution, civil commitment, and loss of parental custody or termination of parental rights.[14]

State policies regarding substance abuse in pregnancy currently vary from harm reduction public heath approaches to punitive laws. At present, Tennessee is the only state that allows assault charges to be filed against pregnant women using illicit substances.[15] Eighteen states consider substance abuse in pregnancy to be child abuse, and 3 consider it to be grounds for civil commitment.[15] The federal Child Abuse Prevention and Treatment Act (CAPTA), initiated in 1974 and reapproved in 2010, mandates that health care providers notify state child welfare agencies of any newborns exposed to prenatal substance abuse.[16] This law is open to state interpretation and implementation, with 18 states requiring reporting of suspected substance abuse in pregnancy, which can be used as evidence in child welfare proceedings.[15] These state laws can include reporting of women on MAT, and are often in place as prerequisites for states to receive public funding for child welfare and substance abuse programs.

Studies have shown these laws to be counterproductive when it comes to reaching pregnant women and engaging them in care.[6,9,14,17,18] When surveyed, women stated that punitive laws would discourage them from seeking care for pregnancy or drug treatment.[17] Punitive laws have not been shown to help the mothers or the infants, are often enforced unequally, and are not designed to ameliorate the factors that contribute to substance abuse recidivism.[6,14] Actions designed to protect the fetus undermine the interconnectedness of maternal and child health, and detract attention and resources away from effective strategies that could help pregnant women and their families.[18]

Incarceration during pregnancy for women with substance abuse disorders is common. As part of the so-called war on drugs, between 1990 and 2009 the number of incarcerated women increased by 153%,[19] and continues to increase as of 2014.[20] Most women are incarcerated for nonviolent crimes such as drug or property offenses.[20] About 6% to 10% of incarcerated women are pregnant,[21] mostly in local jails, which may not have the resources to recognize and treat substance use disorders. Substance use may also continue or begin while in jail.[19] Recognition and treatment of incarcerated, pregnant, opioid-dependent women is essential to increase the likelihood of women entering treatment when released from jail, and avoid the risks of withdrawal, including preterm delivery.[19] Incarcerated opioid-dependent women should be offered the option of methadone or buprenorphine programs; however, not all prison systems have these services available.[19]

Some state laws are protective and prioritize treatment during pregnancy. Nineteen states have programs specifically for pregnant women struggling with substance abuse, whereas 12 states have priority access to state-funded drug treatment programs, and 4 states prohibit state-funded drug treatment programs from discriminating against pregnant women.[15] Pregnant women have a greater need for substance abuse treatment; however, they also have a lower rate of receiving treatment.[22] Expanding available services and reducing the stigma associated with opioid replacement therapy are crucial to ensuring positive health outcomes for mothers and their families.

MEDICAL SYSTEM BARRIERS TO CARE

Discrimination and stigma in the medical system is pervasive toward patients with substance use disorders. Many health care providers have negative views about caring for patients with substance use disorders and often lack the education, training, and support systems to serve them effectively.[23] Adding pregnancy to the mix complicates matters more. Patients can be affected by the lack of empathy of providers, resulting in a lack of empowerment, disconnection from care, and worse treatment outcomes.[23] Despite scientific evidence disproving the teratogenicity of many street drugs, unfair and unproductive treatment of pregnant women struggling with substance use persists.[14] The effects of illicit drugs on fetal development are related primarily to abnormal growth and alterations in neurotransmitter levels and brain development rather than major structural defects.[24] Although opioids are not traditionally viewed as teratogenic, recent epidemiologic studies have showed small increases in odds ratios for certain congenital heart defects,[25] gastroschisis,[25] and spina bifida.[25,26] The significance of these studies is yet to be determined.

The medical system issues facing women with substance use in pregnancy arise from multiple directions. Obstetricians, midwives, and family physicians may be uncomfortable with the topic of substance use, and do not routinely receive training on the screening, recognition, or treatment of substance use disorders. With the current opioid epidemic affecting many communities that previously did not have a significant population of opioid-dependent pregnant women, the knowledge of how to best meet women's needs must become a core aspect of maternity care training. Obstetricians, midwives, and family physicians have an ethical obligation to screen, provide brief interventions, and refer women to substance abuse treatment.[9] Physicians and midwives early in training have more positive or neutral attitudes and believe that they may be able to make a difference in outcomes.[27] Obstetric providers may experience emotional burnout from the high use of resources this population can require, and the sad outcomes that can occur and this can be compounded by a lack of adequate support from substance abuse experts and counselors.[28]

CARE OF OPIOID DEPENDENCY IN PREGNANCY

Physicians caring for opioid-dependent women also encounter special considerations, including complications of drug abuse, management of comorbid illnesses, and management of labor and delivery. Behaviors associated with intravenous drug abuse increase the risk for hepatitis C and human immunodeficiency virus (HIV) from needle sharing, sexually transmitted diseases from trading sex for drugs, and skin infections from injecting drugs.[28] Behaviors associated with drug abuse also put women at greater risk for sexual and physical violence. There are important pregnancy-specific risks to consider, including intrauterine growth restriction and preterm labor.

During labor and postpartum hospitalization, common pain control methods, including intravenous opioids, nitrous oxide, and epidurals, are safe when combined with opioid replacement therapy.[28,29] Opioids may have little analgesic effect for women on buprenorphine and narcotic agonist-antagonist drugs (eg, butorphanol or nalbuphine) can precipitate acute withdrawal and must be avoided in opioid-dependent women. Women may also require higher than average dosing of oral narcotics to achieve adequate pain control after cesarean section.[9,28] Breastfeeding is endorsed by the American Academy of Pediatrics, the American Society of Breastfeeding Medicine, and the American College of Obstetricians and Gynecologists for women who are stable on MAT without illicit substances in urine drug screens.[28–31] Obstetricians, midwives, and family physicians must gain comfort with counseling patients and their families regarding these topics as well as neonatal abstinence syndrome (NAS) during the prenatal period to reduce possible myths and stigma and prepare patients for their delivery experience.

When women who are already established with a medication-assisted treatment provider become pregnant, there are several new considerations. Substance abuse specialists are often uncomfortable with pregnancy, and this discomfort can lead to provider-initiated discontinuation of therapy, patient failure to disclose pregnancy status, and patient avoidance of substance abuse treatment once visibly pregnant because of judgment from other patients receiving therapy. Current literature supports the maintenance of women on medication-assisted treatment with methadone or buprenorphine during pregnancy to avoid growth restriction, preterm labor, and the possible dangers of withdrawal and reduce the risk of relapse.[32] Women with opioid dependence should have the option of either buprenorphine or methadone therapy, however access to either treatment may be unavailable in many areas.[32] Women who are stable on methadone are not usually considered candidates for starting buprenorphine because of the prolonged period of withdrawal required before buprenorphine can safely be started. Opioid detoxification is not recommended as a first-line treatment of opioid addiction in pregnancy because of the high likelihood of the recurrence of opioid use; however, this may be considered in selective situations, such as women returning to communities without access to MAT or women who will be incarcerated.

Methadone has been the standard of care for medication-assisted treatment in pregnancy in the United States since the 1970s.[33] The use of buprenorphine for opioid addiction in pregnancy has increased rapidly since the 2010 Maternal Opioid Treatment: Human Experimental Research (MOTHER) trial showed less severe neonatal withdrawal and equivalent obstetric outcomes.[34–37] The maternal dose of methadone is not related to the incidence or severity of neonatal withdrawal, and therefore methadone should be titrated to alleviate maternal withdrawal symptoms and cravings for illicit drug use.[38–40] Maternal methadone dose should not be decreased during pregnancy, because the higher likelihood of a relapse of opioid abuse increases the incidence of poor pregnancy outcomes, including intrauterine growth restriction and preterm delivery.[29,41] Women who have been on long-term methadone maintenance therapy before conception have more favorable outcomes,[42] presumably because the fetus has not been exposed to the episodic withdrawal that commonly accompanies use of heroin or illicitly obtained prescription opioids.

Infants exposed to buprenorphine in the MOTHER trial required less morphine, had shorter hospital stays, and had a shorter duration of treatment of neonatal withdrawal syndrome compared with infants exposed to methadone, with no significant intrapartum or postpartum outcome differences.[35] There is also no evidence for a dose-response relationship between maternal buprenorphine dose at the time of delivery and neonatal outcomes, including severity of withdrawal or need for pharmacologic treatment.[43] Women who fail buprenorphine treatment may benefit from a supervised daily dosing structure, or may have greater success on methadone.[32] Availability of treatment geographically is another consideration, and expansion of addiction treatment services is needed throughout the United States.

CARE OF THE MOTHER-BABY DYAD DURING NEONATAL WITHDRAWAL

Infants born to mothers with opioid dependence may develop signs of withdrawal, termed NAS. Between 21% and 94% of neonates exposed to opiates in utero develop withdrawal signs and symptoms that are severe enough to warrant pharmacologic treatment.[44–46] Factors that affect the likelihood and severity of NAS include the specific opiate exposure, gestational age, polysubstance abuse, tobacco use, and breastfeeding. An observation period of 96 to 120 hours is typically recommended, during which a scoring system such as the Finnegan scale is used to determine the need for pharmacologic treatment.[44] Oral morphine and methadone are the most commonly used medications, but other agents, such as phenobarbital or clonidine, are sometimes given.[47] Medication must be slowly weaned over several days to weeks, usually in the inpatient setting.

The period of observation and treatment of NAS may occur in a postpartum Mother-Baby unit, nursery, or neonatal intensive care unit. Emerging evidence supports the concept of dyad care, in which mother and infant remain in a private room together throughout the hospitalization.[48] Goals include minimizing ambient noise, staffing by nurses and physicians with special experience in the care of NAS, and providing a comforting environment for mother and baby. One hospital that instituted a rooming-in program decreased the proportion of infants requiring medication from 46% to 27%, reduced average length of stay from 16.9 to 12.3 days, and reduced costs per infant by 50%.[49]

Breastfeeding is also an important element of NAS-related care. Breastfed infants are less likely to require pharmacologic treatment of NAS.[50,51] Levels of both methadone and buprenorphine in breast milk have been shown to be low.[52,53] Instead, breastfeeding benefits for infants exposed to opioids may relate to better tolerability of small frequent feedings, easy digestibility of breast milk, and skin-to-skin contact.[50] In addition, oxytocin produced during letdown promotes mother-infant bonding and may also mitigate against maternal addiction behaviors and stress.[54] However, opioid-dependent women may receive conflicting recommendations from providers regarding the advisability of breastfeeding, and may be discouraged from breastfeeding by family members and partners. Consistent prenatal education regarding this issue and rooming-in practices contribute to more consistent breastfeeding among women.[48] Contraindications to breastfeeding include ongoing use of substances of abuse and HIV infection. Women with hepatitis C infection may breastfeed as long as nipples are not cracked or bleeding. These recommendations are consistent with national guidelines from the American Academy of Pediatrics[31] and the American Academy of Breastfeeding Medicine.[30]

Challenges can arise in neonatal care settings during infant observation and treatment of neonatal abstinence. Obstetricians and other maternity care providers caring for women on MAT need to work collaboratively with pediatricians and family physicians caring for the newborns at risk for NAS. The newborn care team needs to know whether the mother is considered a good candidate for breastfeeding and any concerns regarding ongoing substance abuse. Only about half of neonatal intensive care units in the United States have a written protocol for the diagnosis and management of NAS, leading to differences in care around the country.[55] Structured protocols have been shown to shorten the time of pharmacologic treatment.[56] Despite the benefits of breastfeeding and rooming-in, mothers with economic stress and difficult social situations may not be able to offer this to their newborns. Mothers may face lack of transportation, need to care for other children with limited resources, potential interactions with child protective services, and need to attend daily methadone dosing away from their babies. Maternal medical challenges are also present postpartum, including pain, depression, and relapse. Greater consideration by medical staff of the complex influences of society on the mother-infant dyad will improve outcomes for mothers and babies, and minimize staff burnout.[57]

PSYCHOSOCIAL CHALLENGES

Pregnant women with substance abuse issues often have concurrent mental health issues, and drugs of abuse may cause further deleterious psychiatric effects that prevent or discourage accessing care. Opioid abuse is associated with depressive effects[10] and the highly addictive nature of these substances necessitates a lot of time and effort spent obtaining drugs.[58] Women who use substances in pregnancy often have preexisting psychiatric disorders that prevent them from seeking prenatal care. Women may have difficulty trusting other people, and in particular health care professionals. Women with low socioeconomic status, with or without drug abuse, may think that prenatal care has little or no value.[10] However, when women have had a positive experience with mental health treatment, including for posttraumatic stress disorder, they are more likely to seek prenatal care.[59] If there is a low degree of alliance with their psychiatric health care provider they are less likely to engage in prenatal care.[59]

Women may also be affected by current and historical intimate partner violence. In pregnancy, the prevalence of emotional abuse is 28.4%, physical abuse 13.8%, and sexual abuse 8% in the general population.[60] Abuse before pregnancy, lower education level, unintended pregnancy, low socioeconomic status, and being unmarried, are predictive of abuse in pregnancy.[60] A history of childhood sexual abuse is associated with a significantly increased risk for several psychiatric disorders, intimate partner violence, and substance abuse disorders.[61,62] Women in relationships with ongoing intimate partner violence are less likely to use contraception, including condoms, placing them at risk for unwanted pregnancy and sexually transmitted infections.[63]

Pregnancy ambivalence may also be a concomitant issue. Up to 86% of pregnancies in women using substances may be unintended.[64] This percentage includes 34% mistimed, 27% unwanted, and 26% ambivalent pregnancies.[64] Women may have become pregnant during an abusive relationship, while trading sex for drugs, or during active use of substances. Uncertainty about continuing a pregnancy may lead women to delay prenatal care and sobriety while they are attempting to cope with the unexpected pregnancy. Women may feel additional guilt about terminating a pregnancy on top of their guilt about substance abuse, which may lead to further delays in care. Other women may know they desire a termination but lack access to these services in their geographic area, resulting in continuation of a pregnancy that may not be desired. An understanding of the many intertwining factors facing women who use substances in pregnancy can help providers align with women to ensure the best outcomes for families.

OPTIMIZING THE APPROACH TO CARE

Multidisciplinary models of perinatal substance abuse treatment include prenatal care, opioid replacement therapy, substance abuse counseling, case management services, preparation for parenting, delivery-related services, management of NAS, and primary care for the family, with attention to ongoing developmental care of the child (**Fig. 1**). Programs that incorporate and coordinate this full spectrum of care have shown improved outcomes, including increased rates of program completion and sustained recovery from substance abuse, higher rates of engaging in prenatal care, and greater likelihood of acquiring stable housing,[65] as well as improved birth weights and increased likelihood of mothers retaining custody of their children.[66] Women receiving services via multidisciplinary programs identify respect, caring, and a nonjudgmental approach as central to the therapeutic relationships they have developed with providers and counselors.[65] For women who have experienced childhood abuse and neglect, exploitation via the commercial sex industry, and/or intimate partner violence, these interactions may be the first opportunity to build a sustained healthy relationship with another adult. In addition, loss of their social networks occurs when women choose to avoid contact with friends and family members who continue to engage in substance abuse. Multidisciplinary programs can provide access to a similar group of women who are at varying points along the recovery process, which allows women to share knowledge and experience.[65] Outpatient programs that care for mothers and babies during and after a pregnancy and through the early years of parenting can help prevent adverse childhood events and relapse, and can strengthen young families.[67,68]

Paramount to the success of caring for women with substance abuse disorders in pregnancy is a harm reduction approach and integration of the women's partners and other family members in care.[67] Important aspects of the harm reduction philosophy of care include anticipating and accommodating late arrivals in clinic and missed appointments, using a nonjudgmental style of interaction, positive reinforcement of decreased use as a positive step despite lack of complete abstinence from

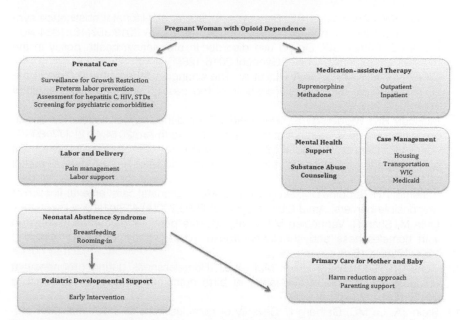

Fig. 1. Considerations for pregnant women and infants in the prenatal, intrapartum, and postpartum periods. STD, sexually transmitted disease. WIC, women infants and children food and nutrition service.

substances of abuse, and following a woman-centered approach. Trauma-informed care acknowledges the role of gender-based and other violence in the development of substance use disorders in women[69] and facilitates trust and respect between women and their providers. Facilitating access to substance abuse treatment for the intimate partners of pregnant women may improve long-term family outcomes, and there is evidence that male partners are overwhelmingly willing to participate in these services when they are available.[70] Although multidisciplinary harm reduction and trauma-informed care are resource intensive and require the ongoing support of a committed group of professionals with skills in obstetric, pediatric, and primary care, as well as addiction medicine, mental health care, and social work, the benefits for this group of underserved women and their children are significant, and form the basis of improved health and social well-being for generations to come.

REFERENCES

1. Hayes MJ, Brown MS. Epidemic of prescription opiate abuse and neonatal abstinence. JAMA 2012;307(18):1974–5.
2. Substance Abuse and Mental Health Services Administration. Behavioral health trends in the United States: results from the 2014 National Survey on Drug Use and Health. 2015. Available at: http://www.samhsa.gov/data/sites/default/files/NSDUH-FRR1-2014/NSDUH-FRR1-2014.pdf. Accessed July 18, 2016.
3. Garg M, Garrison L, Leeman L, et al. Validity of self-reported drug use information among pregnant women. Matern Child Health J 2016;20(1):41–7.
4. Yonkers KA, Howell HB, Gotman N, et al. Self-report of illicit substance use versus urine toxicology results from at-risk pregnant women. J Subst Use 2011;16(5):372–89.

5. Patrick SW, Schumacher RE, Benneyworth BD, et al. Neonatal abstinence syndrome and associated health care expenditures. JAMA 2012;307(18):1934–40.

6. Krans EE, Patrick SW. Opioid use disorder in pregnancy: health policy in the midst of an epidemic. Obstet Gynecol 2016;128(1):4–10.

7. Cicero TJ, Ellis MS, Surratt HL, et al. The changing face of heroin use in the United States: a retrospective analysis of the past 50 years. JAMA Psychiatry 2014;71(7):821–6.

8. McHugh RK, Wigderson S, Greenfield SF. Epidemiology of substance use in reproductive-age women. Obstet Gynecol Clin North Am 2014;41(2):177–89.

9. Jones HE, Deppen K, Hudak ML, et al. Clinical care for opioid-using pregnant and postpartum women: the role of obstetric providers. Am J Obstet Gynecol 2014;210(4):302–10.

10. Schempf AH, Strobino DM. Drug use and limited prenatal care: an examination of responsible barriers. Am J Obstet Gynecol 2009;200(4):412.e1-10.

11. Little M, Shah R, Vermeulen MJ, et al. Adverse perinatal outcomes associated with homelessness and substance abuse in pregnancy. Can Med Assoc J 2005;173(6):615–8.

12. Cutts DB, Coleman S, Black MM, et al. Homelessness during pregnancy: a unique, time-dependent risk factor of birth outcomes. Matern Child Health J 2015;19(6):1276–83.

13. Stein JA, Lu MC, Gelberg L. Severity of homelessness and adverse birth outcomes. Health Psychol 2000;19(6):524–34.

14. Terplan M, Kennedy-Hendricks A, Chisolm MS. Prenatal substance use: exploring assumptions of maternal unfitness. Subst Abus 2015;9:1–4.

15. Guttmacher Institute. Substance abuse during pregnancy. State policies in brief 2016. Available at: https://www.guttmacher.org/state-policy/explore/substance-abuse-during-pregnancy. Accessed July 17, 2016.

16. US Department of Health and Human Services. The child abuse prevention and treatment act: the CAPTA reauthorization act of 2010. Available at: https://www.acf.hhs.gov/sites/default/files/cb/capta2010.pdf. Accessed July 17, 2016.

17. Poland ML, Dombrowski MP, Ager JW, et al. Punishing pregnant drug users: enhancing the flight from care. Drug Alcohol Depend 1993;31(3):199–203.

18. Flavin J, Paltrow LM. Punishing pregnant drug-abusing women: defying law, medicine, and common sense. J Addict Dis 2010;29(2):231–44.

19. American College of Obstetricians and Gynecologists. Committee Opinion 511: Health care for pregnant and postpartum incarcerated women and adolescent females. Obstet Gynecol 2011;118:1198–202.

20. Carson, EA. Prisoners in 2014. US Dept of Justice Bureau of Justice Statistics 2014. Available at: http://www.bjs.gov/content/pub/pdf/p14.pdf. Accessed July 17, 2016.

21. Clarke JG, Hebert MR, Rosengard C, et al. Reproductive health care and family planning needs among incarcerated women. Am J Public Health 2006;96(5):834–9.

22. Terplan M, McNamara EJ, Chisolm MS. Pregnant and non-pregnant women with substance use disorders: the gap between treatment need and receipt. J Addict Dis 2012;31:342–9.

23. van Boekel LC, Brouwers EP, van Weeghel J, et al. Stigma among health professionals towards patients with substance use disorders and its consequences for healthcare delivery: systematic review. Drug Alcohol Depend 2013;131(1–2): 23–35.

24. Behnke M, Smith VC. Prenatal substance abuse: short- and long-term effects on the exposed fetus. Pediatrics 2012;131(3):e1009–24.

25. Broussard CS, Rasmussen SA, Reefhuis J, et al. Maternal treatment with opioid analgesics and risk for birth defects. Am J Obstet Gynecol 2011;204(4):314.e1-11.
26. Yazdy MM, Mitchell AA, Tinker SC, et al. Periconceptional use of opioids and the risk of neural tube defects. Obstet Gynecol 2013;122(4):838–44.
27. Fonti S, Davis D, Ferguson S. The attitudes of healthcare professionals toward women using illicit substances in pregnancy: a cross-sectional study. Women Birth 2016;29(4):330–5.
28. Kremer ME, Arora KS. Clinical, ethical, and legal considerations in pregnant women with opioid abuse. Obstet Gynecol 2015;126(3):474–8.
29. ACOG Committee on Health Care for Underserved Women, American Society of Addiction Medicine. Opioid abuse, dependence, and addiction in pregnancy. Committee opinion no. 524. Obstet Gynecol 2012;119:1070–6.
30. Academy of Breastfeeding Medicine Protocol Committee. Clinical protocol #21: guidelines for breastfeeding and the drug dependent woman. Breastfeed Med 2009;4:225–8.
31. American Academy of Pediatrics. Policy statement; breastfeeding and the use of human milk. Pediatrics 2012;129:e827–41.
32. Holbrook AM. Methadone versus buprenorphine for the treatment of opioid abuse in pregnancy: science and stigma. Am J Drug Alcohol Abuse 2015;41(5):371–3.
33. Finnegan LP. Management of pregnant drug-dependent women. Ann N Y Acad Sci 1978;311:135–46.
34. Jansson LM, Velez M. Neonatal abstinence syndrome. Curr Opin Pediatr 2012; 24:252–8.
35. Jones HE, Kaltenbach K, Heil SH, et al. Neonatal abstinence syndrome after methadone or buprenorphine exposure. N Engl J Med 2010;363(24):2320–31.
36. Jones HE, Johnson RE, Jasinski DR, et al. Buprenorphine versus methadone in the treatment of pregnant opioid-dependent patients: effects on the neonatal abstinence syndrome. Drug Alcohol Depend 2005;79(1):1–10.
37. Lejeune C, Simmat-Durand L, Gourarier L, et al. Prospective multicenter observational study of 260 infants born to 259 opiate-dependent mothers on methadone or high-dose buprenorphine substitution. Drug Alcohol Depend 2006;82(3): 250–7.
38. Cleary BJ, Donnelly J, Strawbridge J, et al. Methadone dose and neonatal abstinence syndrome-systematic review and meta-analysis. Addiction 2010;105(12): 2071–84.
39. McCarthy JJ, Leamon MH, Parr MS, et al. High-dose methadone maintenance in pregnancy: maternal and neonatal outcomes. Am J Obstet Gynecol 2005;193: 606–10.
40. McCarthy JJ, Leamon MH, Stenson G, et al. Outcomes of neonates conceived on methadone maintenance therapy. J Subst Abuse Treat 2008;35(2):202–6.
41. Kraft WK, van den Anker JN. Pharmacologic management of the opioid neonatal abstinence syndrome. Pediatr Clin North Am 2012;59(5):1147–65.
42. Burns L, Mattick RP, Lim K, et al. Methadone in pregnancy: treatment retention and neonatal outcomes. Addiction 2007;102(2):264–70.
43. Jones HE, Dengler E, Garrison A, et al. Neonatal outcomes and their relationship to maternal buprenorphine dose during pregnancy. Drug Alcohol Depend 2013; 134:414–7.
44. Hudak ML, Tan RC. Neonatal drug withdrawal. Pediatrics 2012;129(2):e540–60.
45. Ebner N, Rohrmeister K, Winklbaur B, et al. Management of neonatal abstinence syndrome in neonates born to opioid maintained women. Drug Alcohol Depend 2007;87(2–3):131–8.

46. Logan BA, Brown MS, Hayes MJ. Neonatal abstinence syndrome: treatment and pediatric outcomes. Clin Obstet Gynaecol 2013;56(1):186–92.
47. Kocherlakota P. Neonatal abstinence syndrome. Pediatrics 2014;134:e547–61.
48. Newman A. Rooming-in for infants of opioid-dependent mothers. Can Fam Physician 2015;61(12):e555–61.
49. Holmes AV, Atwood EC, Whalen B, et al. Rooming-in to treat neonatal abstinence syndrome: improved family-centered care at lower cost. Pediatrics 2016;137: e20152929.
50. Welle-Strand GK, Skurtveit S, Jansson LM, et al. Breastfeeding reduces the need for withdrawal treatment in opioid-exposed infants. Acta Paediatr 2013;102: 1060–6.
51. Wachman EM, Byun J, Phillipp BL. Breastfeeding rates among mothers of infants with neonatal abstinence syndrome. Breastfeed Med 2010;5(4):159–64.
52. Lindemalm S, Nydert P, Svensson JO, et al. Transfer of buprenorphine into breast milk and calculation of infant drug dose. J Hum Lact 2009;25(2):199–205.
53. Jansson LM, Choo RE, Harrow C, et al. Concentrations of methadone in breast milk and plasma in the immediate neonatal period. J Hum Lact 2007;23(2): 184–90.
54. Tops M, Koole SL, IJzerman H, et al. Why social attachment and oxytocin protect against addiction and stress. Pharmacol Biochem Behav 2014;119:39–48.
55. Sarkar S, Donn SM. Management of neonatal abstinence syndrome in neonatal intensive care units: a national survey. J Perinatol 2006;26:15–7.
56. Hall ES, Wexelblatt SL, Crowley M, et al. Implementation of a neonatal abstinence syndrome weaning protocol: a multicenter cohort study. Pediatrics 2015;136(4): e803–10.
57. Marcellus L. Neonatal abstinence syndrome: reconstructing the evidence. Neonatal Netw 2007;26(1):33–40.
58. Roberts SC, Pies C. Complex calculations: how drug use during pregnancy becomes a barrier to prenatal care. Matern Child Health J 2011;15:333–41.
59. Bell SA, Seng J. Childhood maltreatment history, posttraumatic relational sequelae, and prenatal care utilization. J Obstet Gynecol Neonatal Nurs 2013;42:404–15.
60. James L, Brody D, Hamilton Z. Risk factors for domestic violence during pregnancy: a meta-analytic review. Violence Vict 2013;28(3):359–80.
61. Jackson A, Shannon L. Factors associated with the chronicity of intimate partner violence experiences among pregnant women in detoxification services. Women Health 2015;55(8):883–99.
62. Nelson EC, Heath AC, Lynskey MT, et al. Childhood sexual abuse and risks for licit and illicit drug-related outcomes: a twin study. Psychol Med 2006;36(10): 1473–83.
63. Maxwell L, Devries K, Zionts D, et al. Estimating the effect of intimate partner violence on women's use of contraception: a systematic review and meta-analysis. PLoS One 2015;10(2):e0118234.
64. Heil SH, Jones HE, Arria A, et al. Unintended pregnancy in opioid-abusing women. J Subst Abuse Treat 2011;40(2):199–202.
65. Racine N, Motz M, Leslie M, et al. Breaking the cycle pregnancy outreach program. J Assoc Research Mothering 2009;11:279–90.
66. Buckley V. Predictors of neonatal outcomes amongst a methadone and/or heroin-dependent population referred to a multidisciplinary perinatal and family drug health service. J Obstet Gynaecol 2013;53:464–70.
67. Ordean A, Kahan M. Comprehensive treatment program for pregnant substance users in a family medicine clinic. Can Fam Physician 2011;57(11):e430–5.

68. Lefebvre L, Midmer D, Boyd JA, et al. Participant perception of an integrated program for substance abuse in pregnancy. J Obstet Gynecol Neonatal Nurs 2010; 39(1):46–52.
69. Torchalla I, Linden IA, Strehlau V, et al. "Like a lots happened with my whole childhood": violence, trauma, and addiction in pregnant and postpartum women from Vancouver's Downtown Eastside. Harm Reduct J 2013;11:1–10.
70. Jones HE, Tuten M, O'Grady KE. Treating the partners of opioid-dependent pregnant patients: feasibility and efficacy. Am J Drug Alcohol Abuse 2011;37(3): 170–8.

Hearing the Silenced Voices of Underserved Women

The Role of Qualitative Research in Gynecologic and Reproductive Care

Angela K. Lawson, PhD[a], Erica E. Marsh, MD, MSCI[b],*

KEYWORDS

- Qualitative research • Underserved women • Gynecology • Fibroids

KEY POINTS

- Patient-centered care requires that health systems understand the unique needs and values of patients.
- Quantitative research designs provide an important but limited understanding of women's health experiences and needs.
- Limited understanding of women's health experiences and needs can lead to the development of ineffective health care strategies and treatment.
- Qualitative research exploring women's health and lived experiences uniquely helps give a voice to the health experiences of underserved women.
- Qualitative research enables the provision of truly patient-centered care and lays the groundwork for inclusive quantitative studies.

INTRODUCTION

Patient-centered care (PCC) is health care that is respectful, compassionate, equitable, transparent, and responsive to patients' needs and values.[1,2] Although the concept of PCC has been academically discussed for many decades,[1] it was not until the Institute of Medicine defined PCC as a primary aim for improvement in health care that the concept seems to have been widely integrated into health systems.[1,2] Since

ª Division of Reproductive Endocrinology and Infertility, Department of Obstetrics and Gynecology, Feinberg School of Medicine, Northwestern University, 676 North Saint Clair Street, Suite 1845, Chicago, IL 60611, USA; ᵇ Division of Reproductive Endocrinology and Infertility, Department of Obstetrics and Gynecology, University of Michigan Medical School, L4000 Women's Hospital, 1500 East Medical Center Drive, Ann Arbor, MI 48109, USA
* Corresponding author.
E-mail address: marshee@med.umich.edu

Obstet Gynecol Clin N Am 44 (2017) 109–120
http://dx.doi.org/10.1016/j.ogc.2016.11.005
0889-8545/17/© 2016 Elsevier Inc. All rights reserved.

obgyn.theclinics.com

that time, predominantly quantitative research has found that PCC is associated with many positive health outcomes, including improved physical and emotional well-being, patient satisfaction, treatment adherence, and patient-physician communication.[1,3,4] However, in order to achieve these positive outcomes, health systems must first understand the unique needs and values of patients; this likely requires the use of qualitative research designs that can inform subsequent quantitative studies. It is therefore vital for health care research to include qualitative analysis of the perspectives and experiences of patients who have historically been overlooked. The purpose of this article is:

1. To describe the strengths and limitations of qualitative approaches and how they differ from the more common quantitative approaches.
2. To describe why this approach is particularly important for underserved communities.
3. To review application of qualitative studies to various populations of underserved women.

Qualitative Versus Quantitative Research Paradigms

Researchers seek to gain knowledge in order to increase insight and solve problems. They may rely on diverse worldviews or paradigms that guide their beliefs about how knowledge is constructed and how it can be discovered. Two common paradigms are the positivist and naturalistic/constructionist paradigms. These paradigms respectively provide the framework for quantitative and qualitative approaches to inquiry.[5] Although each approach provides valuable insight and data, the naturalistic approach to data inquiry often provides the richest understandings of women's lived experiences and health behaviors.

First, within the positivist paradigm, knowledge/reality is thought to be objective, measurable, and cannot be socially constructed. As a result of the fixed nature of reality, study results can be generalized to other people and situations. Positivist researchers frequently conduct studies to test theories or models using a deductive approach. The theory is chosen a priori and then hypotheses are developed to be tested. Research within the positivist paradigm typically takes a quantitative approach to inquiry. Quantitative research methods include the collection of numeric or categorical data either through experiment or survey, which are then statistically analyzed to test the relationship between independent and dependent variables (**Box 1**).[5–7]

In contrast, naturalistic researchers believe that individuals construct knowledge through engagement with others in the world and that knowledge/reality is subjective because the interpretation of data is influenced by the researcher's beliefs. Their approach to data inquiry is inductive and generates a theory or hypothesis following the examination of participant's perspectives. Naturalistic researchers therefore often use qualitative research designs to collect data.[5,7] Three common qualitative research designs are:

1. Phenomenology, which is used to describe the perspectives of people who have experienced a particular phenomenon.
2. Ethnography, which involves the exploration and understanding of a specific culture or group.
3. Grounded theory, which seeks to construct a theory about how individuals work to resolve problems.[8]

When little is known about a phenomenon, qualitative research may lead to increased understanding and the generation of theories of the phenomenon. Quantitative research is therefore guided by the results of qualitative research. Thus,

Box 1		
Underlying assumptions for positivistic and naturalistic research approaches		
Type of Assumption	**Positivist Approach**	**Naturalist/Constructivist Approach**
Research design	Quantitative	Qualitative
Epistemology	Knowledge is uncovered by detached scientific observations	Knowledge is socially constructed through interaction of the researcher with research participants. The values of both the researcher and the research participants contribute to knowledge
	Reality is independent of any opinions of the researcher. The researcher tries to minimize subjectivity and to maximize objectivity	
Ontology	Reality is singular and objective. Reality is constructed based on cause-and-effect inferences	Reality is plural and subjective. Each study participant has a different view on the phenomenon being studied
Methodology	Deductive reasoning	Inductive reasoning
	Statistical hypothesis testing	Theory or hypothesis construction
	Objective and measurable	Subjective and nonmeasurable
	Prediction and estimation	Exploration of participants' experiences
	Identifying associations between variables	Provide rich description of the phenomenon being investigated
	Generalization from samples to population	Generate hypothesis or theory
		Generalization does not matter
	Rule-bound	Context-bound
	Statistical analyses	Content analyses
	Internal and external validity	Credibility, transferability
	Reliability	Dependability, confirmability
	Sample is large or random	Sample size is often small

Modified from Tavakol M, Sandars J. Quantitative and qualitative methods in medical education research: AMEE guide no 90: part I. Med Teach 2014;36:746–56.

although these paradigms are often viewed as competing, they are complementary.[5] Further, the boundary between qualitative and quantitative research is often blurred because quantitative research designs may include inferences about meaning based on the magnitude of study results and qualitative research designs may explore the magnitude of study findings. In addition, most research includes an interplay between inductive and deductive approaches to inquiry.[6]

For centuries, the positivist paradigm and resulting quantitative research has been the predominant approach to data inquiry.[5] However, interest in qualitative research has dramatically increased in the last 40 years. The rapid expansion of interest in qualitative research resulted in increased challenges of the assumptions of qualitative research and led to what is referred to as the (paradigm wars); a war regarding the superiority of quantitative or qualitative research.[7] As a result of this war, and despite the complementary and often blended nature of qualitative and quantitative research, qualitative research has been criticized and devalued.[5] This outcome may contribute to the limited number of qualitative articles that are published, the limited publication of qualitative studies in influential journals, and the lower level of funding for qualitative research compared with quantitative studies.[9,10]

It has been argued that qualitative research designs are not rigorous and the resulting data collected are neither valid nor reliable.[5,7,8] This argument seems to be driven by the inappropriate requirement that qualitative research adhere to the same principles and goals as quantitative research. Where research designs in quantitative research seek to control extraneous variables in the prediction of causal or correlational relationships, replicate statistical findings, and seek exactitude; qualitative research allows for variability and may even seek out the experience of outliers, focuses on naturalistic and unstructured contexts, and may not include a focus on causation and replication. Thus, qualitative research has its own goals and criteria that are vital to understanding the rich lived experiences of individuals.[7,11]

The differences in principles and goals of qualitative and quantitative research are evident not only in research design but also in sample selection, data collection, data analysis, and data interpretation (see **Box 1**). For example, there are sampling differences in qualitative and quantitative research, with sample sizes often being larger and selected more randomly in quantitative research because quantitative researchers often focus on the reduction of sampling error and the power of a study required to detect statistical differences, whereas quantitative researchers may desire nonrandom/purposive sampling in an effort to richly describe the phenomena being studied. Data collection in qualitative research is also appropriately less standardized than is typical in quantitative research. Unlike quantitative research, qualitative research does not rely on tests, questionnaires, structured interviews, or other closed-ended measures. Data collection in qualitative research relies on open-ended protocols.[8,11,12] Further, data collection in qualitative research ends once data saturation is reached; when no more new data are able to be uncovered and additional collected data are redundant.[8,12]

Differences in data analysis and interpretation between quantitative and qualitative research are also apparent. Rather than statistical analysis of quantifiable data and deductive inferences about study results, a common approach to qualitative data analysis is content analysis, which inductively examines and explains shared concepts within the data and groups them in codes and then into broader categories. These categories are labeled and then grouped into themes that illustrate the phenomena being studied.[8,11] Given that the goals of data collection and analyses for quantitative research are often the discovery of quantifiable differences compared with rich descriptions of phenomena respectively, requiring qualitative research to use quantitative statistical analyses would be inappropriate.

Ultimately, both qualitative and quantitative researchers are concerned about the quality of the data generated. However, qualitative researchers describe these concepts using language that differs from that of quantitative researchers. For example, qualitative researchers may use the term credibility instead of internal validity to represent data that are accurate and they may reference the transferability of data, meaning that the study results are generalizable (similar to external validity) to other contexts. Similar to the traditional concept of reliability, qualitative researchers may discuss the dependability of data, which indicates that the same results would be discovered if study participants were reinterviewed. Further, confirmability is similar to quantitative objectivity and reflects that study data reflect study participants' experiences and not researchers' biases (**Box 2**). The rigor of qualitative studies may be ensured via the explicit description of the study design; justification of the use of a qualitative approach to data inquiry; the search for disconfirmatory data; participant review of study findings (member checks); inclusion of participant exemplar statements; as well as description and justification of sample population selection, sample size, and data collection. Further, use of trained interviewers, assessment of coder

Box 2		
Data quality criteria for quantitative and qualitative research		
Data Quality Criteria	**Quantitative Research**	**Qualitative Research**
Confidence in the accuracy of findings	Internal validity	Credibility
Generalizability of findings to other settings	External validity	Transferability
Reproducibility of findings	Reliability	Dependability
Findings are unbiased	Objectivity	Confirmability

reliability, recorded and independently transcribed interview data, and systematic and reproducible data analysis may serve to increase the rigor of a qualitative study.[8,9,12,13]

In addition, unlike quantitative research, the validity of qualitative data is not typically based on statistical analyses but on discussions with study participants, focus groups, or other researchers to confirm the researcher's interpretations. Qualitative data, although often rigorously analyzed thematically through computer software programs, are also not typically analyzed through statistical means but may be analyzed through multiple approaches depending on the phenomena being studied. However, mixed method studies that combine qualitative and quantitative research approaches frequently include both thematic and statistical data analysis and thus may capitalize on the strengths of both data inquiry approaches.[8,9,12,13]

Qualitative Research in Clinical Science

Quantitative research methods do not always provide the best understanding of health behaviors.[7,12] For example, qualitative research may be a more appropriate course of data inquiry when the phenomenon being studied is difficult to quantify, when greater comprehensive understanding of the phenomenon is desired, in order to generate hypotheses as to relationships and causal mechanisms, and to study populations that may be underrepresented in research because of low literacy and/or marginalization.[12,14] Multiple examples exist that highlight the value of qualitative research more than quantitative research. One such study qualitatively examined why participants in a quantitative study of health and behavior change following myocardial infarction reported low attendance rates in a recommended rehabilitation program. Subsequent qualitative interview of these participants revealed that patients had low motivation to make behavioral health changes because they thought that survival following myocardial infarction meant that their medical problems were mild. As a result of the findings of this qualitative study, changes can be implemented to create a new and potentially more effective behavior change rehabilitation program.[15–17] Another example of the incremental benefit of qualitative data beyond that of quantitative data can be seen in a clinical case study of a woman from an underserved population who was gang raped. While meeting with a hospital counselor, the patient was advised to engage in coping strategies that were empirically supported as effective by quantitative research but were largely unavailable or otherwise inappropriate to the patient given her specific life context. Through qualitative data collection, the counselor was able to work to better understand the patient and provide coping strategies that would be uniquely effective for the patient.[18]

In addition to the general added benefit of qualitative research in understanding health behaviors, it has been argued that quantitative research has historically been monocultural, with a focus on homogenous eurocentric populations. Such research has often excluded the experiences of women and minority populations. Qualitative health research that focuses solely on the experiences of women from majority populations also limits understanding of diverse women's experiences. As a result, what is known about health and behavior change may not be generalizable to these populations and may result in the application of ineffective medical interventions and ongoing health disparities for women.[14,19] This possibility applies particularly to women who are also sexual minorities, from low socioeconomic backgrounds, and/or women from racial/ethnic minority groups.

Sexual minorities

Quantitative research confirms that lesbian, bisexual, queer/questioning (LBQ) women and transgender men (individuals who are born biologically female and identify and often present as male) may experience disparate access to and quality of medical treatment, health challenges, discrimination, and harassment.[20–22] Although limited quantitative research has explored the health needs and experiences of LBQ women, less is known about transgender men's health experiences because their experiences are often inappropriately grouped with LBQ women despite sexual orientation and gender identity being different issues.[21] Given the unique health experiences of lesbian, bisexual, transgender, queer/questioning individuals, qualitative research is needed to gain insight into these women's and transgender men's experiences.

Qualitative research on the health needs of LBQ women has found that the use of appropriate language by medical providers is highly important in providing effective care. For example, when caring for a lesbian patient, use of the term social mother or nonbirth mother to describe the female partner of a woman who has given birth may be offensive because it may be seen as minimizing the woman's role as a mother.[23,24] Lesbian/bisexual (LB) women have also described the importance of a supportive clinic environment (eg, use of gender-neutral language on clinic forms, use of supportive language, appropriate emotional support) as well as the inclusion of their partners in their reproductive health care.[25] For example, in a qualitative study by Wojnar and Katzenmeyer[24] (2013) one lesbian woman described her concern about being treated differently by her physician: "Because we were different … I felt I had to be perfect … I dressed neatly and I was really supportive to my partner. I was afraid a nurse or a doctor would come into the room and judge that same-sex couples who decided to have babies are not good to each other or that I don't know how to be a supportive partner in labor or postpartum period."[24] Overall, it seems that providing a supportive environment for LBQ women's reproductive care is vital because LBQ women's negative interactions with their health care providers may play a large role in these women not seeking routine gynecologic care.[22]

Transgender men also have unique gynecologic concerns because they may take testosterone, engage in breast binding, or undergo surgical removal of their breasts, ovaries, and/or uterus. However, limited research has examined transgender men's health experiences or needs. The limited quantitative studies of this patient population have often focused on rates of disease prevalence or reproductive hormone levels. Qualitative research on transgender men's health experiences provides far greater insight into these patient's experiences. For example, one qualitative study of transgender men's gynecologic health needs reveals that, despite not being fond of receiving gynecologic care, transgender men perceive gynecologic care to be important. However, transgender men report experiencing gender dysphoria during gynecologic examinations and often report concern about sharing their identity with their physicians as well as concerns related to clinic forms, which only ask patients to identify their sex and not their gender. As one study participant stated: "More options on the forms means there is room in people's minds."[21]

Additional quantitative research on sexual minority women and transgender men has found that many LB women and transgender men want to become parents.[26,27] Although this is interesting, it does not provide information about the ways in which LB and transgender (LBT) patients experience family building. LBT patients often must pursue medical treatment to begin family building because they require the use of donor sperm, donor egg, and/or gestational surrogacy. Qualitative research specifically examining transgender men's experiences of medically assisted reproduction reveal that, for these patients, lack of acceptance, problematic clinic forms, fear of mistreatment if they revealed their gender identity or advocated for their own care, and even refusal of treatment.[28] Thus, as with LBQ research, research with transgender men indicates that the reduction of barriers in gynecologic care likely involves the use of gender-neutral language on clinic forms or forms that allow transgender men to identify their gender, supportive clinic environments, and acknowledgment of the emotional complexities involved in transgender men's gynecologic care.[21]

Low socioeconomic status

Another group of women whose health experiences are understudied in research are women from low socioeconomic status backgrounds, particularly for low-income housed and homeless women. Limited research has examined these women's gynecologic needs. Quantitative research with this population is difficult given the transient nature of the patient population and the difficulties in accessing large random samples of low-income housed and/or homeless women. What quantitative research exists has shown that these women are at greater risk of certain depressive and anxiety disorders, sexual assault, sexually transmitted diseases, chronic health problems, and unintended pregnancies.[29]

Several qualitative studies of homeless women's health experiences reveal that homeless women are often primarily focused on their own survival and that their health needs were often not a high priority. Further, many homeless women were unable to take advantage of the health care system because of transportation, employment, housing, or childcare concerns, whereas others had low access to health care needs (eg, condoms, feminine hygiene products). Other women did not access health care as a result of low health literacy, particularly as it related to sexually transmitted infections; concern regarding trauma reactions in vaginal examinations; perceived low quality of care; and perceived lack of respect from medical providers, which resulted in some women not disclosing they were homeless.[29–31] For example, in Kennedy and colleagues'[30] (2014) interview study of homeless women, one woman stated, "It's just heavy. Say like you don't know where you're going to be living in the next month, day, year, you know. You can't focus on too much other things. And so if I have to just eliminate a couple of things just to keep my mind focused—children got to school, okay, I might have to go to work, I'm trying to get this housing…you can't stop to take care of your health sometimes. So it's very, very, very hard." Without this understanding of low-income housed and homeless women's lived experiences gleaned through qualitative inquiry, the implementation of gynecologic and other health care that ignored the unique needs of this population would likely prove ineffective.

Racial/ethnic minorities

Despite making up an increasing percentage of the population, the gynecologic challenges of women of African, Asian, and Native American descent, as well as women of Hispanic ethnicity, remain understudied, largely because of challenges in recruitment of these populations to participate in studies. What little research exists with racial/ethnic minority participants highlights the clinical importance of qualitative findings because qualitative studies have provided important perspectives on these women by giving voice to their gynecologic health care experiences and beliefs. Although quantitative studies may tell us the "what" of these populations, qualitative studies help us understand the "why."

For example, quantitative research findings regarding racial/ethnic minority women's gynecologic health has found that African American women (AAW) have a higher mortality from cervical cancer compared with other groups of women; this difference seems to be driven by differences in rates of cervical cancer screening (ie, the "what" is the cause of these differences). However, a qualitative study by Ackerson and colleagues[32] (2010) shows that AAW women who engage in regular screening have supportive mothers and physicians who reinforce the importance of screening and explain the medical reasons for screening (ie, "why" AAW women may not be participating in screening). Thus simply being told to have an annual Pap smear is a less effective mechanism than using family networks and engaged providers who educate patients to effectively encourage AAW women to undergo screening. Similarly, for women of Middle Eastern descent, qualitative research has also found that greater medical explanation of the importance of cervical screening is needed. However, as a result of cultural norms regarding modesty, women of Middle Eastern descent may benefit more from the support and encouragement of their husbands rather than their mothers to undergo cervical screening.[33]

Qualitative research has also highlighted important differences and insights among minority women seeking infertility or pregnancy care. For example, qualitative research has found that Hispanic women may desire that their physicians not only communicate with them in their primary language but that they also desire physicians who act like they are their friends during treatment.[34,35] Qualitative research has also found that different cultural and religious beliefs about infertility may result in increased stigma, fear of interpersonal violence or divorce, and reduced treatment seeking for some women. For these women, physician awareness of and sensitivity to different cultural beliefs about health, improved health education, and inclusion of religious and other supports may play a vital role in encouraging women to seek treatment.[34,36–43] These recommendations are similar to those resulting from qualitative studies of women from racial/ethnic minority groups who historically engage in lower rates of breast cancer screening than white women.[44–48]

The contributions of qualitative research to the gynecologic health of minority women is particularly evident in research focusing on women living with fibroids. Although fibroids have been found to disproportionately affect AAW, research on women's lived experience with fibroids often includes fewer AAW women than white women (eg, see Refs.[49–53]). Quantitative research has identified multiple differences in fibroid characteristics (eg, uterine size and weight, number of fibroids, age at diagnosis, and time between diagnosis and surgery), risk factors (eg, obesity, history of hypertension, family history of fibroids), and potential sequelae (eg, infertility; heavy menses; disruption in physical activities, relationships, and work) between AAW and white women.[54,55] It is likely that the aforementioned differences, as well as other demographic and cultural differences, influence AAW's lived experience with fibroids, thus AAW's voices with regard to fibroids warrant attention.

Results of the few published qualitative studies of women's experiences with fibroids in which most of the participants are AAW have provided a richer understanding of AAW's experiences. In 2015, Ghant and colleagues[56] published one of the first studies that qualitatively examined primarily AAW's perspectives regarding fibroids. This study found that women with fibroids experienced psychological stress (including fear of dying) and a sense of loss of control over their bodies. For example, one woman in the study stated, "I became a little worried because I am like something is wrong with me and I don't understand it. I actually thought at one point … am I dying, God am I dying?" Further, women with fibroids reported a decrease in self-esteem as a result of their fibroids and a desire for greater social support surrounding their experience with fibroids.[56] This study reinforced the need for emotional and psychological support for patients with fibroids; largely minority women.

Another qualitative study of a large number of AAW's treatment seeking behaviors found that women received delayed diagnoses of fibroids because they inaccurately thought their fibroid-related symptoms (eg, abnormal uterine bleeding) were normal and many women had low health literacy about fibroids. The limited health literacy regarding the seriousness of symptomatic fibroids is evident in the statement of one woman in the study who reported, "…my period lasted for 30 days and it was heavy and it was horrible. I was wearing pads like the size that you get in the hospital after you have a baby and I was so used to that happening that at that time I didn't call anybody because you know it was like this is normal."[57] Although some women lacked relevant knowledge about fibroids, others knew something was wrong but actively avoided seeking help for various personal reasons.[57] In addition, one identified qualitative study examined racial/ethnic differences in lived experiences with fibroids. Results of this study by Sengoba and colleagues[58] (2016) confirm the importance of separately examining AAW's perspectives regarding fibroids because AAW in this study reported higher treatment expectations, greater treatment barriers and financial challenges, poorer recovery experiences, and decreased satisfaction compared with other women.[58] Overall, it seems that, among AAW women with fibroids, increased social and emotional support and health literacy education are warranted to improve the gynecologic care of these women.

SUMMARY

Patient-centered care requires that health systems understand the unique needs and values of patients. However, historically, clinical health research has often excluded the experiences of women and minority patient populations. Further, clinical research has often relied on quantitative research strategies; this provides an interesting but limited understanding of women's health experiences and hinders the provision of effective PCC. Therefore, rigorous qualitative research exploring women's health and lived experiences needs to be included, encouraged, and funded in order to enable the provision of high-quality evidence-based health care to women.

REFERENCES

1. Rathert C, Wyrwich MD, Boren SA. Patient-centered care and outcomes: a systematic review of the literature. Med Care Res Rev 2013;70:351–79.
2. Richardson WC, Berwick D, Bisgard J, et al. Crossing the quality chasm: a new health system for the 21st century. Washington, DC: National Academy Press, Institute of Medicine; 2001.
3. Rao JK, Anderson LA, Inui TS, et al. Communication interventions make a difference in conversations between physicians and patients: a systematic review of the evidence. Med Care 2007;45:340–9.
4. Griffin SJ, Kinmonth AL, Veltman MW, et al. Effect on health-related outcomes of interventions to alter the interaction between patients and practitioners: a systematic review of trials. Ann Fam Med 2004;2:595–608.
5. Tavakol M, Sandars J. Quantitative and qualitative methods in medical education research: AMEE guide no 90: part I. Med Teach 2014;36:746–56.

6. Landrum B, Garza G. Mending fences: defining the domains and approaches of quantitative and qualitative research. Qual Psychol 2015;2:199–209.
7. Jackson MR. Resistance to qual/quant parity: why the "paradigm" discussion can't be avoided. Qual Psychol 2015;2:181–98.
8. Tavakol M, Sandars J. Quantitative and qualitative methods in medical education research: AMEE guide no 90: part II. Med Teach 2014;36:838–48.
9. Wisdom JP, Cavaleri MA, Onwuegbuzie AJ, et al. Methodological reporting in qualitative, quantitative, and mixed methods health services research articles. Health Serv Res 2012;47:721–45.
10. McKibbon KA, Gadd CS. A quantitative analysis of qualitative studies in clinical journals for the 2000 publishing year. BMC Med Inform Decis Mak 2004;4:11.
11. Gelo O, Braakmann D, Benetka G. Quantitative and qualitative research: beyond the debate. Integr Psychol Behav Sci 2008;42:266–90.
12. Curry LA, Nembhard IM, Bradley EH. Qualitative and mixed methods provide unique contributions to outcomes research. Circulation 2009;119:1442–52.
13. Devers KJ. How will we know "good" qualitative research when we see it? Beginning the dialogue in health services research. Health Serv Res 1999;34:1153–88.
14. Napoles-Springer AM, Stewart AL. Overview of qualitative methods in research with diverse populations. Making research reflect the population. Med Care 2006;44:S5–9.
15. Wiles R. Patients' perceptions of their heart attack and recovery: the influence of epidemiological "evidence" and personal experience. Soc Sci Med 1998;46: 1477–86.
16. Jolly K, Bradley F, Sharp S, et al. Follow-up care in general practice of patients with myocardial infarction or angina pectoris: initial results of the SHIP trial. Southampton Heart Integrated Care Project. Fam Pract 1998;15:548–55.
17. Jolly K, Bradley F, Sharp S, et al. Randomised controlled trial of follow up care in general practice of patients with myocardial infarction and angina: final results of the Southampton Heart Integrated Care Project (SHIP). The SHIP Collaborative Group. BMJ 1999;318:706–11.
18. Fine M. Coping with rape: critical perspectives on consciousness. Imagin Cogn Pers 1983;3:249–67.
19. Sidani S, Guruge S, Miranda J, et al. Cultural adaptation and translation of measures: an integrated method. Res Nurs Health 2010;33:133–43.
20. Weisz VK. Social justice considerations for lesbian and bisexual women's health care. J Obstet Gynecol Neonatal Nurs 2009;38:81–7.
21. Dutton L, Koenig K, Fennie K. Gynecologic care of the female-to-male transgender man. J Midwifery Womens Health 2008;53:331–7.
22. Hutchinson MK, Thompson AC, Cederbaum JA. Multisystem factors contributing to disparities in preventive health care among lesbian women. J Obstet Gynecol Neonatal Nurs 2006;35:393–402.
23. Brennan R, Sell RL. The effect of language on lesbian nonbirth mothers. J Obstet Gynecol Neonatal Nurs 2014;43:531–8.
24. Wojnar DM, Katzenmeyer A. Experiences of preconception, pregnancy, and new motherhood for lesbian nonbiological mothers. J Obstet Gynecol Neonatal Nurs 2014;43:50–60.
25. Ross LE, Steele LS, Epstein R. Lesbian and bisexual women's recommendations for improving the provision of assisted reproductive technology services. Fertil Steril 2006;86:735–8.
26. Riskind RG, Patterson CJ. Parenting intentions and desires among childless lesbian, gay, and heterosexual individuals. J Fam Psychol 2010;24:78–81.

27. Wierckx K, Van Caenegem E, Pennings G, et al. Reproductive wish in transsexual men. Hum Reprod 2012;27:483–7.
28. James-Abra S, Tarasoff LA, Green D, et al. Trans people's experiences with assisted reproduction services: a qualitative study. Hum Reprod 2015;30:1365–74.
29. Gelberg L, Browner CH, Lejano E, et al. Access to women's health care: a qualitative study of barriers perceived by homeless women. Women Health 2004;40:87–100.
30. Kennedy S, Grewal M, Roberts EM, et al. A qualitative study of pregnancy intention and the use of contraception among homeless women with children. J Health Care Poor Underserved 2014;25:757–70.
31. Oliver V, Cheff R. Sexual health: the role of sexual health services among homeless young women living in Toronto, Canada. Health Promot Pract 2012;13:370–7.
32. Ackerson K. Personal influences that affect motivation in pap smear testing among African American women. J Obstet Gynecol Neonatal Nurs 2010;39:136–46.
33. Khan S, Woolhead G. Perspectives on cervical cancer screening among educated Muslim women in Dubai (the UAE): a qualitative study. BMC Womens Health 2015;15:90.
34. Baxley SM, Ibitayo K. Expectations of pregnant women of Mexican origin regarding their health care providers. J Obstet Gynecol Neonatal Nurs 2015;44:389–96.
35. Nachtigall RD, Castrillo M, Shah N, et al. The challenge of providing infertility services to a low-income immigrant Latino population. Fertil Steril 2009;92:116–23.
36. Becker G, Castrillo M, Jackson R, et al. Infertility among low-income Latinos. Fertil Steril 2006;85:882–7.
37. Fledderjohann JJ. 'Zero is not good for me': implications of infertility in Ghana. Hum Reprod 2012;27:1383–90.
38. Obeisat S, Gharaibeh MK, Oweis A, et al. Adversities of being infertile: the experience of Jordanian women. Fertil Steril 2012;98:444–9.
39. Batool SS, de Visser RO. Experiences of infertility in British and Pakistani women: a cross-cultural qualitative analysis. Health Care Women Int 2016;37:180–96.
40. Ying LY, Wu LH, Loke AY. The experience of Chinese couples undergoing in vitro fertilization treatment: perception of the treatment process and partner support. PLoS One 2015;10:e0139691.
41. Culley L, Hudson N, Rapport F. Assisted conception and South Asian communities in the UK: public perceptions of the use of donor gametes in infertility treatment. Hum Fertil (Camb) 2013;16:48–53.
42. Takahashi S, Fujita M, Fujimoto A, et al. The decision-making process for the fate of frozen embryos by Japanese infertile women: a qualitative study. BMC Med Ethics 2012;13:9.
43. Loke AY, Yu PL, Hayter M. Experiences of sub-fertility among Chinese couples in Hong Kong: a qualitative study. J Clin Nurs 2012;21:504–12.
44. Ogedegbe G, Cassells AN, Robinson CM, et al. Perceptions of barriers and facilitators of cancer early detection among low-income minority women in community health centers. J Natl Med Assoc 2005;97:162–70.
45. Bailey EJ, Erwin DO, Belin P. Using cultural beliefs and patterns to improve mammography utilization among African-American women: the witness project. J Natl Med Assoc 2000;92:136–42.
46. Rodriguez EM, Bowie JV, Frattaroli S, et al. A qualitative exploration of the community partner experience in a faith-based breast cancer educational intervention. Health Educ Res 2009;24:760–71.

47. Ferrante JM, Wu J, Dicicco-Bloom B. Strategies used and challenges faced by a breast cancer patient navigator in an urban underserved community. J Natl Med Assoc 2011;103:729–34.
48. Watson-Johnson LC, DeGroff A, Steele CB, et al. Mammography adherence: a qualitative study. J Womens Health (Larchmt) 2011;20:1887–94.
49. Askew J. A qualitative comparison of women's attitudes toward hysterectomy and myomectomy. Health Care Women Int 2009;30:728–42.
50. Deal LS, Williams VS, Fehnel SE. Development of an electronic daily uterine fibroid symptom diary. Patient 2011;4:31–44.
51. Diaz OV, Guendelman S, Kuppermann M. Subjective social status and depression symptoms: a prospective study of women with noncancerous pelvic problems. Womens Health Issues 2014;24:649–55.
52. Lerner D, Mirza FG, Chang H, et al. Impaired work performance among women with symptomatic uterine fibroids. J Occup Environ Med 2008;50:1149–57.
53. Nicholls C, Glover L, Pistrang N. The illness experiences of women with fibroids: an exploratory qualitative study. J Psychosom Obstet Gynaecol 2004;25: 295–304.
54. Moorman PG, Leppert P, Myers ER, et al. Comparison of characteristics of fibroids in African American and white women undergoing premenopausal hysterectomy. Fertil Steril 2013;99:768–76.e1.
55. Stewart EA, Nicholson WK, Bradley L, et al. The burden of uterine fibroids for African-American women: results of a national survey. J Womens Health (Larchmt) 2013;22:807–16.
56. Ghant MS, Sengoba KS, Recht H, et al. Beyond the physical: a qualitative assessment of the burden of symptomatic uterine fibroids on women's emotional and psychosocial health. J Psychosom Res 2015;78:499–503.
57. Ghant MS, Sengoba KS, Vogelzang R, et al. An altered perception of normal: understanding causes for treatment delay in women with symptomatic uterine fibroids. J Womens Health (Larchmt) 2016;25(8):846–52.
58. Sengoba KS, Ghant MS, Okeigwe I, et al. Racial/ethnic differences in women's experiences with symptomatic uterine fibroids: a qualitative assessment. J Racial Ethn Health Disparities 2016. [Epub ahead of print].

Is There a Shortage of Obstetrician-Gynecologists?

Jody Stonehocker, MD*, Joyce Muruthi, MD, William F. Rayburn, MD, MBA

KEYWORDS

- Demand • Obstetrician-gynecologist • Supply • Workforce

KEY POINTS

- Projections of supply and demand for obstetrician-gynecologists suggest a current minimal or modest shortage that will worsen in the future.
- A modest growth in demand for women's health care will relate to states with population growth (Florida, Texas), where supply is currently less than adequate (rural regions, western United States), and the growing Hispanic population.
- The annual number of ob-gyn residency graduates has increased negligibly, whereas the proportion accepted into fellowships increased steadily, reducing those in general practice.
- The gradual increase in proportion of ob-gyns who are women coincides with desires for more work-life balance and earlier retirement from clinical practice.
- As the supply of advanced practice providers of women's health services grows, the need for more ob-gyns could be less to meet the projected demand.

INTRODUCTION

Training the right number and mix of obstetrician-gynecologists (ob-gyns) is vital to ensuring the nation's goals of access for women to high-quality, affordable health care services. Adult women constitute two-fifths of the US population, and reproductive-age women equal the number of children through early adolescence.[1] Use of women's health care services, the available supply of services, and how care is delivered are determined by several factors: choices made by consumers, practicing women's health care professionals, health care facilities, payers, employers, and federal and state regulatory and payment policies.[1]

Dr W. Rayburn is an unpaid consultant for the American College of Obstetrician Gynecologists on physician workforce issues and strategic planning. Dr J. Stonehocker and Dr J. Muruthi have nothing to disclose.
There are no conflicts of interest in preparing this article.
Department of Obstetrics and Gynecology, University of New Mexico School of Medicine, MSC 10 5580, 1 University of New Mexico, Albuquerque, NM 87131, USA
* Corresponding author.
E-mail address: jstonehocker@salud.unm.edu

Obstet Gynecol Clin N Am 44 (2017) 121–132
http://dx.doi.org/10.1016/j.ogc.2016.11.006
0889-8545/17/© 2016 Elsevier Inc. All rights reserved.

obgyn.theclinics.com

In their capacity of addressing women's health care, ob-gyns play a vital role in achieving these national goals. Having accurate pictures are essential about the current and projected future demand for women's health services and the supply, specialty mix, and characteristics of the ob-gyn workforce. This information is critical for guiding policy and planning initiatives, medical school and residency training priorities, and access to high-quality and affordable care for all women.

COMPLEXITIES OF PHYSICIAN SUPPLY AND DEMAND

Perhaps the best summary of the current and future physician workforce is provided by the Association of American Medical Colleges (AAMC) Center for Workforce Studies.[2] The AAMC engaged IHS Inc (www.ihs.com) to conduct periodic studies that incorporate the latest modeling methods and available data on trends and factors affecting the physician workforce.

Obstetrics and gynecology was viewed as a surgical subspecialty. Although results from the 2016 AAMC update do not focus on ob-gyn specifically, the following were key findings[3]:

- Demand continues to grow faster than supply, leading to a projected total shortfall of between 61,700 and 94,700 physicians by 2025. Projected shortfalls by 2025 range between 14,900 and 35,600 physicians in primary care and between 37,300 and 60,300 in nonprimary care.
- Under virtually all scenarios, the supply of surgical specialists is projected to decline by 2025. The supply of primary care physicians, medical specialists, and other specialists is projected to grow over this period in nearly all supply scenarios.
- For all specialty categories, physician retirement decisions are projected to have the greatest impact on supply, and more than one-third of all currently active physicians will be 65 or older within the next decade.
- Population growth and aging continue to be the primary drivers of increasing demand, with the elderly being expected to experience the greatest growth in demand.
- Expansions in medical insurance coverage due to the Patient Protection and Affordable Care Act (ACA) and the economic recovery have reduced the number of uninsured. This expanded coverage is only projected to increase demand by another 10,000 to 11,000 physicians (1.2%), however.

DEMAND FOR WOMEN'S HEALTH CARE

The demand for women's health care is anticipated to increase with institution of the ACA in 2014. Because of the length of time and expense required to train new physicians, imbalances between the supply and demand for the current women's health care providers is inevitable. Demand determinants involve characteristics of the female population to be served. Economic, cultural, and health risk factors are examples of endpoints to measure in assessing the use and delivery of health care services. One means for quantifying health care demand unique to women is by examining the use of services delivered most often by ob-gyns.

Growth in the US Adult Female Population

Changes in the nation's adult (18 years or older) female population will change over the next 30 years (2015–2045), a period that encompasses the usual professional lifespan of a physician in active practice. A review of US Census Bureau projections reveals that the adult female population is expected to increase by 20.5% from 163.0 million in 2015 to 196.4 million by 2045.[4] Variations in these projections exist, largely being dependent on net immigration, fertility, and mortality rates.

The US adult female population will expand by one million per year between now and 2045. **Fig. 1** displays the growth according to age groups. According to US Census Bureau projections, the working-age female population (18–64 years old) is expected to increase by 10.5 million, whereas its share of the total female population will decline from 61.3% to 56.2%. Women who are 65 or older represent the fastest growing population.[4] By 2045, it is projected that the percentage of women over 65 will be greater than those under 18.

The non-Hispanic white population will peak in 2024 and then decline slowly. A significant increase will be observed among the Hispanic (28.0 million to 50.0 million), black (20.8 million to 26.0 million), Asian (8.6 million to 14.6 million), and American Indian and Alaska Native (1.2 million to 1.4 million) populations. The older population (65 or older) is expected to nearly double and remain predominantly non-Hispanic white (40.7%).

Changes in Health Care Need

Several trends will likely continue in the health care needs of adult women. Examples include longer-acting and reliable contraception, delayed and perhaps lower birth rates, more evidence-based justification for well-woman examinations, and less need for major gynecologic surgery.

Long-acting contraception and lower birth rates

A primary reason for a person to seek initial care from an ob-gyn is for contraception needs. The ob-gyn will have to adapt practice patterns to reflect the trend toward delayed child-bearing and wider access to contraception. The overall birth rate in the United States has steadily declined since 2007, despite the growing reproductive age population.[5] The largest decline in birth rate has been among women less than the age of 30, especially teenagers. Conversely, the birth rate for women over the age of 30 has increased. These observations would be partially explained by greater use of improved contraception, particularly among adolescents.[6] Changes in perceptions of the general public about long-acting, reversible contraception (LARC) methods

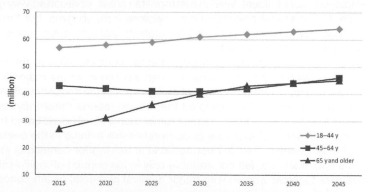

Fig. 1. Projected numbers of adult women in the United States between 2015 and 2045, according to age groups. (*Data from* U.S. Census Bureau, Population Projections, 2012. Available at: https://www.census.gov/population/projections/data/national/2012/summarytables. html. Accessed September 28, 2016.)

and less restrictive criteria for eligibility have led to an increase in use of LARC methods for women aged 15 to 44 from 8.5% to 11.6%.[7]

Well-woman examinations

Periodic assessments, as charted by the Committee on Gynecologic Practice of the American College of Obstetricians and Gynecologists (ACOG), have offered excellent guidelines in providing age-specific preventive screening, evaluation, and counseling on a yearly basis (as recommended by the College) or as appropriate.[8] A final report of the Well-Woman Task Force (Components of the Well-Woman VISIT), a collaborative initiative involving 14 national medical and provider societies and hosted by ACOG, became available in April 2014.[9] The primary question deals with the growing body of evidence that does not support the need for periodic routine examinations. If yearly Pap tests and pelvic and breast examinations are unnecessary, why have a yearly examination? Fewer women may not seek routine annual preventive care or counseling by an ob-gyn or may feel more comfortable receiving this reshaped well-woman care from their family physician or internist.

Fewer major gynecologic surgeries

Obstetric and gynecologic surgeries constitute up to one-fourth of all inpatient surgical procedures in the United States.[10] The number of cesarean deliveries increased 1.5-fold between 1979 and 2006.[10] During that same period, the number of hysterectomies, sterilizations, oophorectomies, prolapse, and incontinence procedures decreased by nearly half. This significant decline reflects an increased rate of minimally invasive surgery and advances in medical interventions that preclude a need for major surgery.

Providing Care Beyond the Reproductive Years

As the population ages, a growing group of women no longer needs care focused on reproduction or contraception. Do women aged 45 and older still seek care from their ob-gyn even though they do not need pregnancy care? Results from 2 major ambulatory medical care surveys revealed that only 12% to 16% of all women aged 45 or older obtained care from ob-gyns either alone or with family physicians and general internists.[11] Most visits to an ob-gyn office were for a checkup or for diagnosis or treatment rather than ongoing care of a chronic medical condition. Women were more likely to see an ob-gyn, rather than a family physician, if they were non-Hispanic white, married, employed, more affluent, lived in metropolitan areas, or reported very good to excellent care. Fewer sought preventive care services from ob-gyns, but those who did were seeking screening or intervention for menopausal symptoms, cervical cancer, breast cancer, and osteoporosis.

The population of older Americans is expected to represent 20% of the total US population in the next 50 years, and older women will comprise the majority of that group.[4] A survey of a representative group of ob-gyns about the frequency of care provided to women 65 years or older revealed that 86.4% reported that they cared for older women.[12] A higher proportion of female rather than male ob-gyns cared for older patients. About half reported adequate or comprehensive training in the overall general health of older patients. Few felt comfortable in training for conditions involving other systems and, therefore, felt comfortable only in the context of multidisciplinary collaborative care for older women with major medical or mental health concerns.

Projected Demand for Women's Health Services

The only known study to estimate the demand for women's health care by 2020 was reported by Dall and colleagues[13] using 2012 national utilization standards. The report incorporated the most current national data resources to design a simulation model to create health and economic profiles for a representative sample of women from each state. Demand was determined using equations about projected use of ob-gyn services.

The national demand for women's health care was forecast by Dall and colleagues[13] to grow by 6% by 2020. Most (81%) ob-gyn–related services were for women of reproductive age (18–44 years old). Growth in demand was forecast to be highest in states with the greatest population growth (Florida, Texas), where supply is currently less than adequate (rural regions and western United States), and among Hispanic women. This increase in demand by 2020 will translate into a greater need for physicians or advanced practice providers, that is clinically equivalent to 2090 full-time ob-gyns.

SUPPLY OF OBSTETRICIAN-GYNECOLOGISTS

The number of active physicians describing ob-gyn as their primary interest has doubled since 1975, despite remaining about 5% of all active physicians.[1] This growth is less than for physicians in pediatrics, family medicine, and internal medicine, yet similar to those practicing psychiatry. The number of ob-gyns per 10,000 adult women in the general US population increased minimally from 8.7 in 1980 to 10.8 in 2016.[1] Many ob-gyns are viewed as coordinators of care for reproductive age (15–44) women. However, most become specialists and serve as collaborators with family physicians and internists beyond the reproductive years.[11]

The supply of ob-gyns is dependent on several factors, which include, but are not limited to, trends in residency and fellowship training, millennial work hours, migration patterns, retirement, and growth of advanced practice providers.

Residency Positions

Concerns have been raised that the number of residents in ob-gyn training programs is inadequate to meet demands of the growing adult female population in the United States. A review of data from the National Residency Match Program revealed that the number of accredited programs declined minimally (from 257 in 1992 to 242 in 2015), whereas the number of first-year positions increased only slightly (from 1110 in 1992 to 1255 in 2015).[1,14]

The minimal increase of first-year residency positions in ob-gyn was outpaced by a steady growth in the US adult female population. Using data from the population division of the US Census Bureau disclosed a growth in the adult female population by 9.6% from 89.5 million to 98.1 million during this same period.[4] This difference can be viewed in the context that for every first-year residency position, there were 89,452 adult women in 1992 and 98,076 in 2015.[15] This increase will continue as the number of residency positions is expected to not increase appreciably in the future.

Fellowship Training

Most ob-gyns in general practice choose not to provide the entire breadth of core components required for certification from the American Board of Obstetrics and Gynecology (ABOG). As with residents in other specialties, more ob-gyn graduates are pursuing subspecialty fellowship training, adding to the complexities of workforce planning.[16] More than one-fourth of resident graduates pursued a variety of accredited and nonaccredited fellowship programs, as shown in **Table 1**. The proportion accepted into fellowships increased steadily in all accredited subspecialties

Table 1 Percentages of obstetrician-gynecologists resident graduates who pursued further training in different fellowships, 2016	
Family planning	1.9%
Female pelvic medicine and reconstructive surgery	3.4%
Gynecologic oncology	4.5%
Maternal-fetal medicine	7.6%
Minimally invasive gynecologic surgery	5.0%
Pediatric and adolescent gynecology	0.3%
Reproductive endocrinology and infertility	4.0%
Total	26.7%

From Rayburn WF, Gant NF, Gilstrap LC, et al. Pursuit of accredited subspecialties by graduating residents in obstetrics and gynecology, 2000-2012. Obstet Gynecol 2012;120:619–25; with permission.

(gynecologic oncology, maternal-fetal medicine, and reproductive endocrinology and infertility [REI]) from 7.0% in 2000 to 19.5% in 2012.[16]

The numbers of newly ABOG-approved female pelvic medicine and reconstructive surgery programs and positions have increased significantly and are now similar to numbers in REI.[16] Furthermore, numbers of resident graduates accepted into non-ABOG or non–Accreditation Council for Graduate Medical Education programs such as minimally invasive gynecologic surgery and family planning and less formal postgraduate training in infectious disease, hospitalist care, global health, breast disease, ultrasonography, women's health research, and critical care are smaller and less available. Clearly, there are more options for graduates to specialize. This movement toward subspecialization will require monitoring due to a concern that fewer graduates pursue general obstetrics and gynecology, obstetrics only, or gynecology only.

Millennial Work Hours

The Millennial generation was born between 1980 and 2000 to Baby Boomer parents. They represent young physicians, many of whom view their work and work achievement as being less central to their lives. They are more inclined to "work to make a living" and value specialties that offer a more controllable lifestyle.[17] Ob-gyn has been ranked among the "noncontrollable" lifestyle specialties, especially among those aged 50 or less.[18] Many Millennials desire more part-time work, but do not have this option and are prone to be less satisfied professionally.

In addition, the Millennial generation has been generally characterized as having higher levels of narcissism, which can lead to a higher likelihood of unmet expectations with their careers and overall lower levels of satisfaction.[19] Younger ob-gyns are at risk for lower levels of career satisfaction with less control over their life balance.[18] Burnout may result, which impacts the quality of care physicians provide, physician turnover, and overall quality of the health care system.[20,21] Although this is very important to consider, caution about overgeneralizing is necessary, and more rigorous research is encouraged to adequately represent ob-gyns.

Female Obstetrician-Gynecologists

More than half of all ACOG Fellows and Junior Fellows in practice are women (**Fig. 2**). That proportion is projected to be two-thirds by 2030 as more male Fellows retire.[1] Compared with male ob-gyns, female ob-gyns are younger and more likely to work part time.[18,22] This desire to work part time is likely influenced by delaying

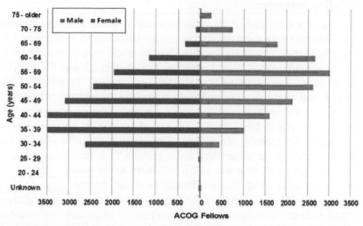

Fig. 2. Numbers of ACOG Fellows and Junior Fellows in active practice in 2016, by age range and gender.

child-bearing until training is completed and balancing career building with raising young children.[23]

Married female physicians with children spend more time on parenting and domestic duties than male physicians.[24] Although physicians report high satisfaction with the relationships they have with their children, ob-gyns are the least likely to believe that their career had a positive impact on the relationships they developed with their children.[25] The inability to balance work and home responsibilities is associated with female surgeons reporting a moderate or higher likelihood of planning to reduce their clinical work hours or leave their current practice in the next 24 months.[26]

Maldistribution and Migration Patterns

An uneven geographic distribution of physicians is common and has important implications for patient access to routine and specialized care. The distribution of the ACOG Fellows and Junior Fellows in practice is very uneven.[27] Approximately half (1550, 49%) of the 3143 US counties lacked an ob-gyn in 2010. More than 10 million women (8.2% of all women) lived in those predominantly rural counties, many of which were designated as Health Professional Shortage Areas.[27] This maldistribution could worsen if graduating residents cluster in urban areas and as demand for women's health services increases.[13,28]

Local shortages can result from physician migration. An average of 6% of all practicing ob-gyns moves across counties per year.[28] Approximately one-third relocated (usually once or twice) over a recent 10-year period (2005–2015).[28] Migration was more common among general ob-gyns, compared with those who either practiced gynecology or obstetrics only.[28]

Migrations have been predominantly to counties that were urban or had a lower percentage of the population in poverty.[28] More than half (58%) of all relocations were within the same state, often in adjacent counties. Net migration was most positive in Florida, California, and Washington and most negative in Michigan, Pennsylvania, and New York. Observing this trend will contribute to a better understanding about the uneven national distribution of ob-gyns.

Attrition Including Retirement

Attrition from practice is typically from either retirement, either voluntary or involuntary, or death. No published data exist about mortalities for ob-gyns in practice. Mortalities by age and sex from the Centers for Disease Control and Prevention indicate that people in professional occupations have lower mortalities through age 65 compared with the national average. Johnson and colleagues[29] estimated age-adjusted mortalities for professional and technical occupations to be approximately one-fourth lower than national rates for men and 15% lower for women.

Retirement of ob-gyns is becoming a matter of increasing concern in light of an expected shortage of practicing physicians. One-third of ob-gyns are aged 55 years or older, which is similar to other physician groups.[30] A customary age range of retirement from ob-gyn practice would be 59 years to 69 years (median 64 years). **Fig. 3** displays the median and interquartile range of retirement ages of physicians in different specialties. Male and especially female ob-gyns retire at slightly younger ages than those in other medical specialties. This trend is especially important, because women occupy a growing proportion of the ob-gyn workforce. Subspecialists in board-accredited fellowships (gynecologic oncology, maternal fetal medicine, and REI) averaged to be slightly older at retirement.[31]

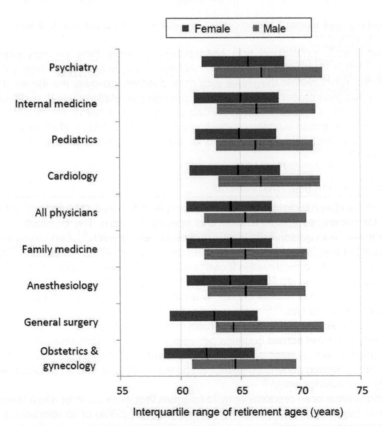

Fig. 3. Interquartile and median ages of retirement from active practice for physicians in different specialties, by gender. (*From* Rayburn WF, Strunk AL, Petterson SM. Considerations about retirement from clinical practice by obstetrician-gynecologists. Am J Obstet Gynecol 2015;213(3):336; with permission.)

The large cohort of Baby Boomer physicians approaching retirement (approximately 15,000 ob-gyns) deserves tracking, as investigations of integrated women's health care delivery models are being conducted. Relevant considerations would include strategies to extend the longevity of those considering early retirement or desiring part-time employment. Likewise, volunteer work in underserved community clinics, with or without medical students or residents, offers continuing personal satisfaction for many retirees.

Physician Re-entry

The number of ob-gyns leaving their practice and wishing to return is unknown but likely very small. This number may increase, however, with more female ob-gyns in the workforce.[1] Constructing a re-entry education program for any physician includes the following challenges: determining which candidates are most eligible; individualizing the curriculum based on their needs; evaluating a trainee's progress and competency in completing the program; and realizing the cost of individualized training.[32] A continuing medical education model can only be undertaken at ob-gyn residency programs that have experienced educators and sufficient clinical and surgical material to not detract from the training of residents and fellows. Indeed, reports of a small number of ob-gyn re-entry programs already exist.[32,33]

Advanced Practice Providers

A growing number of advanced practice providers could theoretically reduce the cost of medical care and need for additional ob-gyns. More than half of all ob-gyn offices currently employ providers such as nurse practitioners (NPs), certified nurse midwives (CNMs), and physician assistants (PAs).[34] Studies over the past 30 years have found that these frontline practitioners perform as well, if not better, than physicians for many nonoperative routine services.[35]

Growth in the numbers of NP and PA training programs and graduates has been remarkable this past decade, whereas the number of CNM graduates has increased only slightly.[35] Percentages of all active NPs and PAs who work with ob-gyns are unclear but currently estimated to be 9% and 2%, respectively.[1] More graduates are expected as more move away from traditional primary care. Whether ob-gyns and other surgical specialties can absorb many advanced practice providers is unclear. To the extent that the supply of nonphysician clinicians of women's health services grows faster than 6%, the need for more ob-gyn physicians could be less than the projected 6% growth in demand between 2010 and 2020.[13]

SUMMARY

This special report for *Obstetrics and Gynecology Clinics of North America* is intended to answer the question, "Is there a shortage of obstetrician-gynecologists?" Findings were based on certain assumptions that the current national supply of ob-gyns supply is adequate, yet there are insufficient data to either support or refute this. This report took into consideration both demand for and supply of ob-gyns and advanced practice providers in women's health care. Such forecasts require taking into account the current demographics of the provider workforce, numbers and characteristics of graduates, hours worked, desire for work-life balance, and retirement.

Projections of supply and demand suggest a current minimal or modest shortage of ob-gyns that will worsen in the future. In percentage terms, the shortfall is not as great as other surgical specialties, reflecting a modest growth in demand over the supply of ob-gyns and the ability to augment staffing with other types of providers. The supply of ob-gyns is unlikely to increase as much as the demand drivers (eg, population projections) and the more rapid pace in health care delivery. Differences in projections highlight the importance of continually monitoring the projections of supply by incorporating the latest trend in supply with demand determinants, the latest research on care delivery models (eg, Accountable Care Organizations), changing technology, and economic conditions.

Uncertainties exist about how emerging care delivery models and changing care practices will affect ob-gyn supply and women's health care demand and how clinicians and care settings will respond to economic and other trends. This dilemma underscores the need for ongoing research on potential implications of the evolving health care systems. Examples of future research would involve several of the following directions:

1. Pursuit of subspecialty training by ob-gyn resident graduates;
2. Whether younger ob-gyns will continue to have similar work-life balance expectations as older cohorts;
3. How nonphysician staffing patterns will evolve;
4. Effects from different payment models (eg, Medicaid, ACA);
5. Distribution of ob-gyns and relocation patterns; and
6. How ob-gyn retirement or part-time patterns will change, based on economic factors, work satisfaction, trends in women's health, and cultural norms about retirement.

REFERENCES

1. Rayburn WF. The obstetrician-gynecologists workforce in the United States: facts, figures, and implications 2nd edition. Washington, DC: Am College Obstet Gynecol; 2017.
2. Dill MJ, Salsberg ES. The complexities of physician supply and demand: projections through 2025. Washington, DC: Association of American Medical Colleges; 2008.
3. 2016 update. The complexities of physician supply and demand: projections from 2014 to 2025. Final report. Washington, DC: IHS Inc; 2016.
4. Table 3-1 Percent distribution of the projected population by selected age groups and sex for the United States: 2015 to 2060 (NP2012-T3L U.S. Census Bureau, Population Division). Available at: https://www.2census.gov/programs-surveys/popest/. Accessed on September 28, 2016.
5. Martin JA, Hamilton BE, Osterman MJ. Births in the United States, 2015. NCHS data brief, no 258. Hyattsville (MD): National Center for Health Statistics; 2016.
6. American College of Obstetricians and Gynecologists. ACOG Practice Bulletin No. 121: Long-acting reversible contraception: implants and intrauterine devices. Obstet Gynecol 2011;118(1):184–96.
7. Kavanaugh ML, Jerman J, Finer LB. Changes in use of long-acting reversible contraceptive methods among U.S. women, 2009-2012. Obstet Gynecol 2015; 126:917–27.
8. Committee on Gynecologic Practice. Committee opinion No. 534: well-woman visit. Obstet Gynecol 2012;120:421–4.
9. Conry J, Brown H. Well-woman task force: components of the well-woman visit. Obstet Gynecol 2015;126:697–701.
10. Oliphant SS, Jones KA, Wang L, et al. Trends over time with commonly performed obstetric and gynecologic inpatient procedures. Obstet Gynecol 2010;116:926–31.

11. Raffoul M, Rayburn WF, Petterson S, et al. Preferences of specialties for office based care by women 45-64. J Womens Health 2016. [Epub ahead of print].
12. Rayburn WF, Raglan GB, Herman CJ, et al. A survey of obstetrician-gynecologists regarding their care of women 65 years or older. J Geriatr Med Gerontol 2015;1:2–7.
13. Dall TM, Chakrabarti R, Storm MV, et al. Estimated demand for women's health services by 2020. J Womens Health 2013;22:643–8.
14. The Match. National Resident Matching Program. Results and Data. 2016 Main Residency Match. April 2016. Available at: http//www.nrmp.org. Accessed September 15, 2016.
15. Stonehocker J, Murray-Krezan C, Rayburn W. Residency positions in obstetrics and gynecology and growth of the U.S. adult female population, 1992 to 2015. Obstet Gynecol 2016;127:83s–4s.
16. Rayburn WF, Gant NF, Gilstrap LC, et al. Pursuit of accredited subspecialties by graduating residents in obstetrics and gynecology, 2000-2012. Obstet Gynecol 2012;120:619–25.
17. Twenge JM, Campbell SM, Hoffman BJ, et al. Generational differences in work values: leisure and extrinsic values increasing, social and intrinsic values decreasing. J Manage 2010;36:1117.
18. Anderson BL, Hale RW, Salsberg E, et al. Outlook for the future of obstetrician gynecologist workforce. Am J Obstet Gynecol 2008;199(1):88.e1-8.
19. Twenge JM, Foster JD. Birth cohort increases in narcissistic personality traits among American college students, 1982-2009. Soc Psychol Personal Sci 2010; 1:99–106.
20. Shanafelt TD, Balch CM, Bechamps GJ, et al. Burnout career satisfaction among American surgeons. Ann Surg 2009;250:463–71.
21. Keeton K, Fenner DE, Johnson TR, et al. Predictors of physician career satisfaction, work-life balance, and burnout. Obstet Gynecol 2007;109:949–55.
22. Dorsey ER, Jarjoura D, Rutecki GW. The influence of controllable lifestyle and sex on the specialty choices of graduation. U. S. medical students, 1996-2003. Acad Med 2005;80:791–6.
23. Alonso-Basanta M. Work/life balance: a tale of the blue collar father and the white collar daughter. JAMA Oncol 2015;1:1223–4.
24. Jolly S, Griffith KA, DeCastro R, et al. Gender differences in time spent on parenting and domestic responsibilities by high-achieving young physician-researchers. Ann Intern Med 2014;160:344–53.
25. Shanafelt TD, Hasan O, Hayes S, et al. Parental satisfaction of U.S. physicians: associated factors and comparison with the general U.S. working population. BMC Med Educ 2016;16:229.
26. Dyrbye LN, Freischlag J, Kaups KL, et al. Work-home conflicts have substantial impact on career decisions that affect the adequacy of the surgical workforce. Arch Surg 2012;147:933–9.
27. Rayburn WF, Klagholz JC, Murray-Krezan C, et al. Distribution of American College of Obstetricians and Gynecologists Fellows and Junior Fellows in practice in the United States. Obstet Gynecol 2012;119:1017–22.
28. Xierelli IM, Mivet MA, Rayburn WF. Relocation of obstetrician-gynecologists in the United States, 2005-2015. Obstet Gynecol, 2017, in press.
29. Johnson NJ, Sorlie PD, Backlund E. The impact of specific occupation on mortality in the U.S. national longitudinal mortality study. Demography 1999;36(3):355–67.
30. Rayburn WF, Strunk AL, Petterson SM. Considerations about retirement from clinical practice by obstetrician-gynecologists. Am J Obstet Gynecol 2015;213(3): 335.e1-4.

31. Holbrook B, Petterson S, Rayburn W. Retirement ages of maternal-fetal medicine physicians. Am J Perinatol 2016. [Epub ahead of print].
32. Rayburn W, Quintana A, Cosgrove E, et al. Facilitating physician relicensure and reentry into clinical practice: collaboration between a state medical board and a medical school. J Med Res 2016;102:18–22.
33. Varjavand N, Pereiva N, Delvadia D. Returning inactive obstetrics and gynecology physicians to clinical practice: the Drexel experience. J Contin Educ Health Prof 2015;35:65–70.
34. Rayburn WF, Tracy EE. Changes in practice of obstetrics and gynecology. Obstet Gynecol Surv 2015;71:1–7.
35. Waldman R, Powell Kennedy H. Collaborative practice in obstetrics and gynecology. Obstet Gynecol Clin North Am 2012;39:323–44.

Index

Note: Page numbers of article titles are in **boldface** type.

A

Affordable Care Act
   access to care related to, 46–48
   groups most affected by, 50
   impact on family planning, 46–48
African American women
   obesity/overweight in, 58–59
Anticontraceptive politics
   in family planning, 48–49

B

Bisexual
   defined, 72

C

Childbearing
   acknowledging different values about
      in reassessing unintended pregnancy, 32–33
Chronic Care Model
   as postpartum weight intervention, 62, 66
COMPARE-UF registry, 88–89
Continuity of care
   establishing
      in reassessing unintended pregnancy, 32
Contraception
   counseling related to
      in reassessing unintended pregnancy, 34–35
Counseling
   contraception-related
      in reassessing unintended pregnancy, 34–35
Cultural competence
   ensuring
      in improving racial and ethnic disparities, 7
Culture
   as factor in family planning, 45–46

D

Depression
   postpartum
      among sexual minorities, 73–74

Obstet Gynecol Clin N Am 44 (2017) 133–141
http://dx.doi.org/10.1016/S0889-8545(16)30106-1
0889-8545/17

obgyn.theclinics.com

Disparity(ies). *See* Health disparities; Racial disparities; *specific types,*
    e.g., Ethnic disparities
DPP
    in obesity prevention, 66–67

E

Education
    patient-related
        in improving racial and ethnic disparities, 7
    sexuality
        unintended pregnancy effects of, 43–44
Ethnic disparities
    in fibroids, 82–88 *See also* Fibroid(s), racial and ethnic disparities in
    in health and health care, **1–11**
        causes of, 2–5
        future directions in, 5–7
        health care system and institutional level factors in, 4–5
        national impact of, 1–2
        patient-level factors in, 2–4
        provider-level factors in, 4
        research related to, 5
        strategies for improvement in, 5–7
            diversifying health care workforce and ensuring cultural competence, 7
            patient education, 7
            promoting research, 6–7
            raising awareness, 5–6
    in quality of care in obstetrics, **13–25** *See also* Quality of care, in obstetrics,
        disparities in
Ethnicity
    defined, 1
    disparities related to *See* Ethnic disparities

F

Family planning, **41–56**. *See also* Unintended pregnancy
    Affordable Care Act effects on, 46–48
    anticontraceptive politics in, 48–49
    culture and, 45–46
    facilitators in, 50–52
    hospital mergers and, 49–50
    introduction, 41–43
Fibroid(s), **81–94**
    background of, 81–82
    prevalence of, 81
        racial and ethnic disparities in, 82, 89
    racial and ethnic disparities in, 82–88
        disease severity, 83
        earlier onset, 82–83
        growth and regression, 84
        interplay of, 91

prevalence, 82, 89
reproductive outcomes, 87–88, 90
rural/urban, 90–91
socioeconomic status, 89–90
surgical outcomes, 87
symptom severity, 83–84
treatment differences, 85–90
    COMPARE-UF registry on, 88–89
treatment of, 81–82
    options in, 88–89
    racial and ethnic disparities in, 85–90

H
Health
    racial and ethnic disparities in, **1–11** *See also* Ethnic disparities, in health and health
        care; Racial disparities, in health and health care
Health care
    racial and ethnic disparities in, **1–11** *See also* Ethnic disparities, in health and health
        care; Racial disparities, in health and health care
    women's
        demand for
            obstetrician-gynecologists shortage related to, 122–125
Health care disparities
    among sexual minorities, **71–80** *See also specific types and* Sexual minorities, health
        care disparities among
    in reassessing unintended pregnancy
        recognize and address, 37
Health care quality
    defined, 14–15
Health care workforce
    diversification of
        in improving racial and ethnic disparities, 7
Health disparities
    defined, 1–2, 15–16
    national impact of, 1–2
Health equity
    defined, 15–16
Hospital mergers
    family planning effects of, 49–50
Housing, food, and transportation insecurities
    of pregnant women with substance abuse
        PCC in addressing, 96–97
Hysterectomy
    for fibroids, 81–82

L
Leiomyoma(s), **81–94**. *See also* Fibroid(s)
Lesbian
    defined, 72

Lesbian, gay, bisexual, and transgender (LGBT) community
    health care disparities in, 72
        health care access, 75
        interventions for, 75–76
        introduction, 71–73
        mental health, 73–74
        PPD in, 73–74
        preventive health care services, 75
        sexual health, 74
        unmet medical needs, 75
Let's Move
    in obesity prevention, 66
LGBT community. See Lesbian, gay, bisexual, and transgender (LGBT) community

    M

Media
    unintended pregnancy effects of, 44–45
Medical needs
    unmet
        of sexual minorities, 75
Medical system barriers to care
    for pregnant women with substance abuse
        PCC in addressing, 98–99
Mental health
    among LGBT community, 73–74
Myoma(s), **81–94**. See also Fibroid(s)

    N

National Survey of Family Growth (NSFG)
    on unintended pregnancy rates, 41
Neonatal withdrawal
    care of mother-baby dyad during
        PCC in addressing, 100–101
NSFG. See National Survey of Family Growth (NSFG)

    O

Obesity
    in African American women, 58–59
    postpartum-related
        interventions for, **57–69** See also Postpartum weight interventions
    prevention of
        initiatives in, 66–67
Obstetrician-gynecologists
    shortage of, **121–132**
        advanced practice providers, 129
        attrition including retirement, 128–129
        complexities of physician supply and demand, 122
        demand for women's health care, 122–125

changes in health care need, 123–124
growth in US adult female population, 122–123
projected demand for women's health services, 124–125
providing care beyond reproductive years, 124
fellowship training, 125–126
female obstetrician-gynecologists, 126–127
introduction, 121–122
maldistribution and migration patterns, 127
millennial work hours, 126
physician re-entry, 129
residency positions, 125
Opioid dependence
pregnant women with
barriers for
PCC in addressing, **95–107** See also Pregnant women with substance abuse,
barriers for, PCC in addressing
Overweight
in African American women, 58–59
postpartum-related
interventions for, **57–69** See also Postpartum weight interventions

P

Patient-centered care (PCC)
in addressing barriers for pregnant women with substance abuse, **95–107** See also
Pregnant women with substance abuse, PCC in addressing barriers for
described, 109–110
Patient education
in improving racial and ethnic disparities, 7
Patient-provider relationship(s)
in reassessing unintended pregnancy
complexities of, 31
Patient trust
earning
in reassessing unintended pregnancy, 32
PCC. See Patient-centered care (PCC)
Perinatal care
disparities in
outcomes-related, 18–19
Postpartum
as critical phase of woman's lifespan, 58
defined, 57
Postpartum depression (PPD)
among sexual minorities, 73–74
Postpartum weight interventions
developing and implementing
theoretical frameworks for, 62–66
Chronic Care Model, 62, 66
RE-AIM framework, 62
evidence for, 59–62
future research on, 66

Postpartum (*continued*)
    initiatives to prevent obesity, 66–67
    leveraging opportunities for, **57–69**
    policy implications for, 66
PPD. *See* Postpartum depression (PPD)
Pregnancy
    in obese/overweight women
        prevalence of, 57
    unintended *See* Unintended pregnancy
Pregnant women with substance abuse
    background of, 95–96
    epidemiology of, 95–96
    PCC in addressing barriers for, **95–107**
        background of, 95–96
        care of mother-baby dyad during neonatal withdrawal, 100–101
        epidemiology of, 95–96
        housing, food, and transportation insecurities, 96–97
        medical system barriers to care, 98–99
        opioid dependency during pregnancy, 99–100
        optimizing approach to care, 102–103
        psychosocial challenges, 101–102
        societal stigma and criminalization, 97–98
Psychosocial challenges
    of pregnant women with substance abuse
        PCC in addressing, 101–102

Q

Quality of care
    defined, 14–15
    in obstetrics
        disparities in, **13–25**
            discussion, 20–22
            indicators of, 20
            introduction, 13–14
            outcomes-related, 18–19
            terminology related to, 15–16
        measurement of, 16–18
Queer
    defined, 72

R

Race
    defined, 1
    disparities related to *See* Racial disparities
Racial and ethnic minorities
    hearing silenced voices of
        qualitative research on, 115–117
Racial disparities
    in fibroids, 82–88 *See also* Fibroid(s), racial and ethnic disparities in

in health and health care, **1–11**
  causes of, 2–5
  future directions in, 5–7
  health care system and institutional level factors in, 4–5
  national impact of, 1–2
  patient-level factors in, 2–4
  provider-level factors in, 4
  research related to, 5
  strategies for improvement in, 5–7
    diversifying health care workforce and ensuring cultural competence, 7
    patient education, 7
    promoting research, 6–7
    raising awareness, 5–6
in quality of care, **13–25** See also Quality of care, in obstetrics, disparities in
Raising awareness
  in improving racial and ethnic disparities, 5–6
Reach, efficacy and effectiveness, adoption, implementation, and maintenance (RE-AIM) framework
  as postpartum weight intervention, 62
RE-AIM framework. See Research, efficacy and effectiveness, adoption, implementation, and maintenance (RE-AIM) framework
Relationship(s)
  therapeutic
    in reassessing unintended pregnancy, 32–33
Reproductive autonomy
  in reassessing unintended pregnancy, 37
Reproductive preferences
  in reassessing unintended pregnancy, 33–34
Research
  promoting of
    in improving racial and ethnic disparities, 6–7

S
Sexual health
  among sexual minorities, 74
Sexuality education
  unintended pregnancy effects of, 43–44
Sexual minority(ies)
  defined, 72
  health care disparities among, **71–80**
    health care access, 75
    interventions, 75–76
    introduction, 71–73
    mental health, 73–74
    PPD, 73–74
    preventive health care services, 75
    sexual health, 74
    unmet medical needs, 75
  hearing silenced voices of
    qualitative research on, 114–115

Sexual orientation
    defined, 72
Silenced voices of underserved women
    hearing of, **109–120** *See also* Underserved women, silenced voices of, hearing of
Societal stigma and criminalization
    of pregnant women with substance abuse
        PCC in addressing, 97–98
Socioeconomic status
    as factor in race/ethnicity disparities in fibroids, 89–90
    of underserved women
        qualitative research on, 115
Substance abuse
    pregnant women with
        barriers for
            PCC in addressing, **95–107** *See also* Pregnant women with substance abuse, barriers for, PCC in addressing

T

Trust
    patient
        earning
            in reassessing unintended pregnancy, 32

U

Underserved women
    silenced voices of
        hearing of, **109–120**
            introduction, 109–110
            low socioeconomic status, 115
            PCC in, 109–110
            qualitative research in clinical science, 113–117
            qualitative *vs.* quantitative research paradigms in, 110–113
            racial and ethnic minorities, 115–117
            sexual minorities, 114–115
Unintended pregnancy. *See also* Family planning
    defined, 28
    described, 28
    introduction, 41–43
    as marker in clinical encounter
        concerns about using, 29–31
    measuring of
        utility of, 28
    media effects on, 44–45
    NSFG on rate of, 41
    persons affected by, 29
    prevalence of, 29, 41–43
    reassessing, **27–40**
        adopt reproductive justice framework in, 37
        complexities of patient-provider relationship in, 31

develop therapeutic relationship in, 32–33
direct contraception counseling in, 34–35
explore patient-centered approaches to optimize reproductive preferences in, 36
future research in, 35–36
increase access to care in, 36–37
inquire about reproductive preferences in, 33–34
introduction, 27–28
policy implications in, 36–37
practical, patient-centered approach to optimizing reproduction choices in, 31–35
recognize and address health care disparities in, 37
redefine measures and outcomes in, 36
support reproductive autonomy in, 37
sexuality education effects on, 43–44
Unmet medical needs
of sexual minorities, 75

W

Weight
postpartum
interventions for, **57–69** See also Postpartum weight interventions
Women who have sex with women
defined, 72

Moving?

Make sure your subscription moves with you!

To notify us of your new address, find your **Clinics Account Number** (located on your mailing label above your name), and contact customer service at:

Email: journalscustomerservice-usa@elsevier.com

800-654-2452 (subscribers in the U.S. & Canada)
314-447-8871 (subscribers outside of the U.S. & Canada)

Fax number: 314-447-8029

Elsevier Health Sciences Division
Subscription Customer Service
3251 Riverport Lane
Maryland Heights, MO 63043

*To ensure uninterrupted delivery of your subscription, please notify us at least 4 weeks in advance of move.

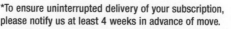

ELSEVIER

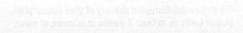

Printed and bound by CPI Group (UK) Ltd, Croydon, CR0 4YY

03/10/2024

01040393-0012